Core Glossary H
核心词汇手册

注：核心词汇手册中部分例句来自《牛津高阶英汉双语词典》（第七版），具体页码在例句后括号内注明。

Nouns（名词）

A

abdomen 腹部

abdominal breathing 腹式呼吸

abdominal muscles 腹部肌肉，腹肌

abdominal region 腹部区域，腹区

acidity 胃酸过多

adrenal gland 肾上腺

advanced stage This man was diagnosed with an advanced stage of cancer.（晚期）
这个男的被诊断为癌症晚期。

air He kicked that football into the air.（空中，天空）
他把那个足球踢到空中。
Spring is very much in the air.（空气）
空气中弥漫着春的气息。（又译为：春意盎然。）

anchor   Lift your upper back and legs off the floor, using your sitting bones as the anchor.（可靠或主要的支撑）

上背部和双腿抬离地板，使用坐骨作为支点。

angle   Bend your knees to form a right angle.（角度）

屈膝成直角。

ankle   脚踝

ankle joint   踝关节

anxiety   We must clearly know how to deal with anxiety in our daily life.（焦虑）

我们必须清楚地知道如何应对日常生活中的焦虑。

arch   足弓

Achilles tendon   跟腱

area   The tumor has already spread to other areas of his body.（区域，部位）

肿瘤已经扩散到他身体的其他部位了。

arm   胳膊

armpit   腋窝

arthritis   关节炎

Aṣṭāṅga Vinyāsa Yoga   阿斯汤加瑜伽

asthma   哮喘

awareness   Bring awareness to your breath.（意识，觉知）

将意识带到你的呼吸上。

B

baby   This baby girl is so cute!（婴儿）

◆ What we need is the strength of steel, but with steel's flexibility—not like crude iron, which is very very strong and hard but breaks.

这个女婴好可爱！

back 背部（人体部位），背面

backache 背部疼痛

balance They work together to strive for the balance of ecology.（平衡，均衡）

他们通力合作为生态平衡而努力。

ball (of the foot) 跖骨球

base Sacrum is located at the base of the spine.（基底，底面，底部）

骶骨位于脊柱的末端。

belly Inhale, belly out; exhale, belly in.（腹部）

吸气，腹部隆起；呼气，腹部内收。

biceps 二头肌

big toe 大脚趾

bird A little bird rested on my balcony.（鸟）

一只小鸟停在我的阳台上。

benefit The Cobra pose can be of benefit to those that have back problems.（利益，益处）

眼镜蛇式对于背部有问题的人群有益。

bladder 膀胱

blanket 毯子

bloating Bloating usually occurs due to indigestion.（发肿，膨胀）

胀气的出现通常是因为消化不良。

blood circulation A sedentary lifestyle can decrease your blood circulation.（血液循环）

久坐不动的生活方式会使你的血液循环变慢。

◆我们需要的是钢的强度，但又要有钢的韧性——不像生铁那样，无比结实又坚硬，但会断裂。

boat   We can go there by boat.（船）

　　　　我们可以坐船去那儿。

body   身体

bow   He killed that bird with his bow and arrow.（弓）

　　　　他用弓箭杀死了那只鸟。

brain   大脑

branch   Some branches should be cut off.（树枝）

　　　　有些枝条应当被砍掉。

breast   乳房

breath   You can actually control your own breath.（呼吸，气息，一口气）

　　　　实际上你可以控制自己的呼吸。

breathlessness   Heart failure can cause fatigue and breathlessness.（呼吸急促，气喘）

　　　　心衰能够引起疲劳和呼吸困难。

breathing   Her breathing is slow and deep.（呼吸）

　　　　她的呼吸缓慢而深长。

bridge   They decide to build a bridge next month.（桥）

　　　　他们决定下个月建一座桥。

bronchitis   支气管炎

butterfly   I have never seen butterflies in winter.（蝴蝶）

　　　　我从来没在冬天见过蝴蝶。

buttock   臀部

◆ We can achieve steadiness through meditation on the infinite—anything great, huge, well-settled and well-established.

C

calf 小腿肚

calf muscle 腓肠肌

camel 骆驼

cancer 癌症

cardiovascular system 心血管系统

cat 猫

caution Yoga practitioners should be fully aware of the contraindications and cautions of the yoga poses they practise.〔（对危险或风险的）警告，告诫〕
瑜伽习练者应当充分了解他们所练习的瑜伽体式的禁忌及注意事项。

cawing If you listen carefully, you will notice there are at least 5 different notes in birds cawing.（鸦叫声，呱呱叫）
如果你仔细听，你会发现这些鸟鸣声中至少有5个不同的调。

ceiling Lift your head up towards the ceiling.（天花板）
抬头向上，朝向天花板。

centre Focus on the centre of your eyebrows.（中心）
关注眉心。

cervical spine 颈椎

cervical vertebrae 颈椎

chair She is sitting in my chair.（椅子）
她正坐在我的椅子上。

◆我们可以通过冥想于无限——任何伟大的、巨大的、安定的、稳固的事物——来达到稳定。

change A lot of changes have taken place in this small town.（改变，变化）

这个小镇发生了很多变化。

cheek 面颊

chest 胸

chin 下巴

circulatory system 循环系统

clavicle 锁骨

clothes Your clothes were left in that closet.（衣服）

你的衣服落在那个壁橱里了。

cobra Aren't you scared of cobras?（眼镜蛇）

你难道不怕眼镜蛇吗?

coccyx 尾骨，尾椎

cold 感冒

collarbone 锁骨

concentration Yoga is not a game; it requires a great deal of concentration.（专心，专注）

瑜伽不是游戏；它需要你全神贯注地去做。

constipation 便秘

contact Please avoid close contact with others when you have a flu.（接触）

当你患流感时，请避免与他人密切接触。

contraindication Yoga teachers should clearly know the contraindications of the yoga poses they teach.（禁忌证）

◆ If the body is still, it is easy to make the mind still.

瑜伽老师应当清楚地知晓他们所教授的瑜伽体式的禁忌。

coordination　Yoga can very well improve your coordination.〔（身体各部位的）协调能力〕

瑜伽能够很好地提升你的协调能力。

corner　I hit my knee on the corner of the table.（角）

我的膝盖撞到桌子角上了。(p.144)

coronary artery diseases (CAD)　冠状动脉疾病，冠心病

corpse　My favorite pose is Corpse pose because it's so relaxing.（尸体）

我最喜欢的体式是挺尸式，因为它太令人放松了。

count　Raise both legs and hold for a count of 10.（数数，点数）

抬起双腿，保持这一姿势直至数到10。

cow　奶牛，母牛

crocodile　鳄鱼

crow　Crow pose is an advanced yoga pose, but still you could try it.（乌鸦）

乌鸦式是一种高级瑜伽体式，但你仍然可以尝试一下。

cushion　You may put a cushion under your head.（软垫，坐垫）

你可以在头部下方放一个垫子。

D

daily life　We are faced with many challenges in our daily life.（日常生活）

我们在日常生活中面临许多挑战。

◆如果身体是静止的，那么让头脑静止也就容易了。

degree The right foot pointed outward at an angle of 90 degrees.
〔（指角度、经纬度）度〕
右脚以90度角指向外侧。

deltoid 三角肌

depression 抑郁，抑郁症

diabetes 糖尿病

diaphragm 横膈膜

diarrhea 腹泻，痢疾

digestive organ 消化器官

digestive system 消化系统

direction She walked in the direction of a newly opened yoga studio.
（方向）
她朝一家新开的瑜伽馆走去。

distance The yoga studio is within walking distance of my house.
（距离，间隔）
瑜伽馆离我家很近，走几步路就到了。

dizziness 头晕

dog 狗

duodenal ulcers 十二指肠溃疡

E

eagle You could imagine yourself turning into an eagle when you are in Eagle pose.（鹰）
当你在做鹰式的时候，你可以想象自己变成了一只鹰。

ear 耳朵

◆ Through the body we can put a brake on the mind.

earth You could feel the earth shake as the truck came closer.（土地，陆地）

卡车开近时你会感觉到地面在震动。

edge See that the inner edges of your feet are parallel.（边缘）

保证双脚内缘平行。

elasticity Yoga can help retain the elasticity of your skin.（弹性，灵活性）

瑜伽能够帮助保持皮肤弹性。

elbow 手肘

elbow joint 肘关节

endocrine system 内分泌系统

energy Teaching yoga sometimes can be really energy-consuming.（能量，精力）

教瑜伽有时真的很消耗能量。

equestrian This teacher is qualified for teaching equestrian skills.（骑马，骑马者）

这位老师有资格教授马术。

excretory system 排泄系统

exhalation Hold your breath for a count of 5 after your exhalation.（吸入，吸气）

呼气之后，屏住呼吸数到5。

eye 眼睛

eyebrow 眉毛

eye pillow 眼枕

◆通过身体，我们可以在思想上刹车。

F

face   脸

faith   Blind faith may cause a man to go astray.（信仰，信念）
盲目的信仰会使人误入歧途。

fat   If you want to control your weight, you should cut the amount of
fat in your diet.（脂肪，肥肉）
如果你想控制自己的体重，那么你应当减少饮食中的脂肪
含量。

fatigue   Yoga can effectively reduce fatigue and stress.（疲劳，疲乏）
瑜伽能够有效地减轻疲劳与压力。

feeling   How could you say I don't care about your feelings?（感情）
你怎么能说我不在乎你的感受呢?

femur   股骨

fever   发热，发烧

fibula   腓骨

finger   手指

fingernail   手指甲

finger pad   指肚

fingertip   手指尖

fish   He caught a fish and gave it to me as a gift.（鱼）
他捉到一条鱼并将它送给我当礼物。

fist   He raised a clenched fist.（拳头）
他举起了握紧的拳头。

flatulence   胀气

◆ When we take a vow we should stick to it. There will be ample tests to
tempt us to break it.

flesh   Tigers are flesh-eating animals.（肉，肉体）

　　　　虎是食肉动物。(p.774)

flexibility   Some people want to develop the flexibility of their bodies by practising yoga.（灵活性，弹性）

　　　　有些人想要通过练习瑜伽增强身体的柔软度。

floor   Lie on the floor.（地板，地面）

　　　　躺在地板上。

flow   You may feel the flow of energy when you are close to nature. 〔（液体，气体或电）流动〕

　　　　当你接近大自然的时候，你会感受到能量的流动。

Flow Yoga   流瑜伽

flu   流感

foot   Stand with your feet slightly apart.（脚，复数feet）

　　　　双脚微微分开站立。

　　　　One foot is equal to 30.48 centimetres.（英尺）

　　　　一英尺等于30.48厘米。

folding chair   折叠椅

forearm   小臂

forefinger   食指

forehead   额头

forward bend   Many people make mistakes when doing seated forward bend.（前屈）

　　　　许多人在做坐立前屈时会出错。

fragrance   This perfume gives off a sweet fragrance.（香味，芬芳）

　　　　这个香水散发着甜香的气味。

◆我们一旦发了誓就应该坚持。会有诸多的考验诱使我们打破它。

frog　青蛙

front　Yoga teacher usually demonstrate in the front of the classroom.
（前面的）

瑜伽老师通常在教室前面做示范。

functioning　Chanting can clear your mind and improve brain functioning.（运作，功能）

念诵能够清除杂念，提升大脑功能。

G

gallbladder　胆囊

gastric complaints　胃部不适

gastritis　胃炎

gastrocnemius　腓肠肌

gastrointestinal ulcer　消化道溃疡

gaze　He met her gaze.

他与她凝视的目光相遇。(p.844)

gluteus maximus　臀大肌

grassland　Practising yoga on grassland would be unique experience.
（草原，草地）

在草地上练瑜伽将是一种独特的体验。

grip　Suddenly she lost her grip on the yoga strap.（紧握，抓住）

突然她紧攥着瑜伽伸展带的手松开了。

groin　腹股沟

ground　Don't lie on the ground.（地面，土地）

不要躺在地上。

◆ By regulating the prana, we regulate our minds, because the two always go together.

H

hair　头发

half　She cut that melon in half and shared it with her child.（一半，半场，半程）

她把那个瓜切成两半，和孩子一起吃。

hammock　吊床

hamstring　腘绳肌腱

hand　手

happiness　To find happiness, you have to turn inward.（幸福，快乐）

要找到幸福，你得转向内在。

Haṭha Yoga　哈达瑜伽

head　头部

headache　头痛

heart　心脏

heartburn　胃灼热，烧心

heart disease　心脏病

heart problem　心脏问题

heaviness　You may notice the heaviness of your breath.（沉重）

你可能会注意到自己呼吸沉重。

heel　脚跟

height　BMI is determined by your body weight and height.（高度）

身体质量指数是由你的体重和身高决定的。

hemisphere　Australia is located in the southern hemisphere.（半球）

澳大利亚位于南半球。

◆通过调节prana（普拉那，生命之气），我们调节了我们的思想，因为这两者总是相辅相成的。

hernia　疝气

herniated cervical disc　颈椎间盘突出症

herniated disc　椎间盘突出

hero　Who is your hero?
谁是你的英雄?

high blood pressure　高血压

hinge　Use your hips as a hinge to bend forward.（枢纽，转折点）
以你的髋部为折点前屈。

hip　髋，臀

hip flexor　髋屈肌

hip joint　髋关节

hold　Make sure you've got a steady hold on the camera.（抓，握）
一定要拿稳相机。(p.975)

horizon　The sun sank below the horizon.（地平线，视野）
太阳落到地平线下。(p.987)

humerus　肱骨

hunchback　驼背

I

image　The image of that little dog was fixed in her mind.〔影，（头脑里的）形象〕
那只小狗的形象深深地印在她的脑子里。

impression　His words left an everlasting impression on my mind.
（印记，印象）
他的话在我心上留下了不可磨灭的印记。

◆ Without much prana, we can never give anything to anybody, just as only a fully-charged battery can give power, never a weak one.

incision The doctor will make a tiny incision in your abdomen.
（切口）

医生会在你的腹部切个小口。

indigestion 消化不良

inflammation 发炎，炎症

inhalation With an inhalation, raise your hands overhead, palms
facing forward.（吸入，吸气）

随着一次吸气，双手高举过头顶，掌心向前。

injury A few villagers sustained serious injuries in the earthquake.
（损害，受伤）

有几个村民在地震中受了重伤。

insomnia 失眠

instep 脚背

Integral Yoga 整合瑜伽

integumentary system 皮肤系统

intercostal muscles 肋间肌

internal organ 内脏，内脏器官

intestinal tuberculosis 肠结核

instruction Please follow my instructions.（指令，教导）

请跟随我的口令。

irregular periods 月经不规律

ischial bursitis 坐骨滑囊炎

issue Obesity has become a serious health issue nowadays.（问题）

现如今肥胖已经成了一个严重的健康问题。

◆没有太多的生命之气，我们就永远不能给予任何人任何东西，就像只有充满电的电池才能提供能量，而电量不足的电池则不能。

item This is the most expensive item in this collection. 〔一件商品
（或物品）〕
这个是这套收藏品中最贵的一件。

Iyengar Yoga 艾扬格瑜伽

J

joy She shouted with joy when she finished all her tasks. （快乐，
欢喜）
当她完成所有的任务后，高兴地叫了起来。

K

Kids Yoga 儿童瑜伽

knee 膝

kneecap 膝盖骨，髌骨

knee injury 膝关节损伤

knuckle 指关节

L

lap She put the baby on her lap. 〔（人坐着时的）大腿面〕
她将宝宝放在自己腿上。

large intestine 大肠

late-stage 晚期

latissimus dorsi 背阔肌

leaf There was a drop of dew on the lotus leaf. （叶子）
荷叶上有一颗露珠。

◆ Control and discipline are very necessary in our lives.

leg 腿

length He measured the length and width of the classroom.（长度）

他测量了教室的长度和宽度。

level Straighten your arms and hold your thumbs in front of your face at eye level.（水平，水平高度）

手臂伸直，大拇指置于面前与视线水平等高。

lever You can use the lever rule to calculate.（杠杆）

你可以使用杠杆定律进行计算。

ligament She has torn a ligament.（韧带）

她的韧带撕裂了。

lightness Try to feel the lightness of your body when you are in headstand.（轻盈）

当你在头倒立体式中的时候，试着去感受身体的轻盈。

lip 唇

limb 肢体

little finger 小指

little toe 小脚趾

liver 肝脏

locust Locusts are pests.（蝗虫）

蝗虫是害虫。

lord *The Lord of the Rings* is a fantasy novel.（主人，统治者）

《指环王》是一部奇幻小说。

low blood pressure 低血压

lower extremities 下肢

lower jaw 下颌骨

◆控制和自律在我们的生活中是非常必要的。

lower leg　小腿

lumbago　腰痛

lumbar disc herniation　腰椎间盘突出症

lumbar lordosis　腰椎前凸

lumbar vertebrae　腰椎

lumbosacral region　腰骶部

lung　肺

lymphatic system　淋巴系统

M

mandible　下颌骨

meditation　What is your purpose of practising meditation?（冥想，静坐）

你练习冥想的目的是什么?

meniscal tears　半月板撕裂

menopause　Menopause is the period of time when women gradually stop menstruating.（更年期）

更年期是女性逐渐停经的时期。

menstrual cramps　经期痉挛，痛经

menstrual discomfort　经期不适

menstrual disorders　月经失调，经期紊乱

menstrual flow　月经

menstruation　月经

metacarpal　掌骨

metatarsal　跖骨

◆ First we learn to control the physical body, then the movement of the breath, then the sense, and finally the mind.

metre   She is 1.65 metres tall.（米）

　　　　她身高1.65米。

middle   You may practise in the middle of the classroom.（中间，

　　　　中央）

　　　　你可以到教室中间来练习。

middle finger   中指

midline   The seven chakras are located along the midline of human

　　　　body.（中线，中间线）

　　　　七脉轮沿人体中线分布。

mid-stage   中期

mind   Various kinds of thoughts kept running through my mind when

　　　　I meditated.（头脑，思想，思维）

　　　　在我冥想的时候，各种念头不断地在我脑海闪现。

Mindfulness Meditation   正念冥想

minute   See you in a minute!（分钟，片刻）

　　　　　一会儿见！

moment   Everyone listens attentively at this moment.（片刻，时刻）

　　　　　此刻，每个人都聚精会神地听着。

moon   She was thrilled to see such a big bright moon in the sky.（月亮）

　　　　看到天空中如此大的一轮明月，她很兴奋。

mountain   Imagine you are as steady as a mountain when you're in

　　　　Mountain pose.（高山，山岳）

　　　　当你在做山式时，想象自己就像一座山一样稳定。

mouth   嘴巴

◆首先我们学会控制身体，然后是呼吸的运动，然后是感觉，最后是
头脑。

movement   You may feel the gentle movement of your abdomen as you breathe.〔（身体部位的）运动，动作〕
你可能会感受到腹部随着呼吸微微起伏。

muscle   肌肉

muscular system   肌肉系统

N

name   What's the full name of it?（名称，名字）
它的全称是什么？

nausea   恶心

navel   肚脐

neck   颈部

nerve   This breathing technique can help soothe your nerves.（神经）
这种呼吸技巧能够帮助舒缓你的神经。

nervous system   神经系统

night   I usually work more efficiently at night.（夜晚）
我通常在晚上工作效率更高。

nose   鼻子

nostril   鼻孔

O

object   I would like to choose a burning candle as the object of meditation.（物体，客体）
我想选用一支燃烧的蜡烛作为冥想的对象。

◆ The mind is a veil woven of thoughts. It has no substance by itself.

observation　As soon as he entered the classroom, he started his careful observation of the teacher's demonstration.（观察）

他一进到教室就开始认真观察老师的示范。

osteoporosis　骨质疏松症

outline　From here you could see the outline of that bridge.（轮廓）

从这儿你能够看到那座桥的轮廓。

outside　You should check the inside and outside of that house before you buy it.（在……外面）

在你买房之前应该将那个房子里里外外检查一遍。

oxygen　Some breathing techniques can help you breathe in more oxygen.（氧气）

有些呼吸技巧能够帮助你吸入更多氧气。

P

pain　I have a pain in my wrists.

我手腕疼。

pancreas　胰腺

palm　手掌

palpitation　心悸

Parkinson's disease　帕金森病

Partner Yoga　双人瑜伽

patella　膝盖骨，髌骨

pattern　Strictly follow this pattern and that's all you should do.（模式）

你只要严格遵循这个模式就可以了。

pectoralis　胸肌

◆思想是由念头编织而成的面纱。它本身是没有实质的。

pebble　She put several pebbles in the flower pot.（鹅卵石）

她在花盆里放了几颗鹅卵石。

pelvic floor　骨盆底

pelvic region　骨盆区

pelvis　骨盆

peptic ulcer　消化性溃疡

perineum　会阴

plow　犁

point　In that prone pose, eight points of your body touch the floor and hence the name Eight-limbed Salutation.（点）

在那个俯卧体式中，你身上的八个点触地，因此名叫八体投地式。

pose　What is your favorite yoga pose?（姿势，姿态）

你最喜欢的瑜伽体式是什么？

posture　Maintaining good posture can bring you confidence.（姿势，身姿）

保持良好的体态能为你带来自信。

portion　Yoga occupies a small portion of your life even if you practise it 1 hour everyday.（部分）

即使你每天练习瑜伽1小时，瑜伽也只占据你人生中一小部分时光。

position　Make sure your sit in a comfortable position.〔（坐、立的）姿态，姿势〕

确保你的坐姿舒适。

◆ If the senses are allowed to see outside, they try to grasp pictures of the outside world. If they are turned inward, they will see the purity of the mind and won't take the color of the world outside.

practice　You need regular yoga practice.（练习）

你需要规律的瑜伽练习。

practitioner　A good yoga teacher must be, first of all, a good yoga practitioner.（习艺者，习练者）

一个好的瑜伽老师首先得是一个好的瑜伽练习者。

prayer　We believe in the power of prayer.（祈祷）

我们相信祈祷的力量。

pregnancy　Women had better practise yoga under the supervision of a qualified teacher during pregnancy.（怀孕，孕期）

孕期女性最好在有资质的老师的监督指导下练习瑜伽。

Prenatal Yoga　孕期瑜伽

present tense　You may use present tense to describe facts.（现在时态）

你可以使用现在时态描述事实。

pressure　Don't put all the pressure on your knees or wrists.（压力）

不要把所有压力都放到你的膝盖或手腕上。

problem　Go find a doctor to help you when you have a health problem.（问题，难题）

当你有健康问题时，去找医生帮助你。

process　It's only the beginning of a long process.（过程）

它只是一个漫长过程的开端。

psoas　腰肌

pubis　耻骨

pushing force　推力

◆如果允许感官向外看，它们就会试图抓取外界的图片。如果它们转向内在，则将看到心灵的纯洁，而不会沾染外界的颜色。

Q

quadriceps　四头肌

R

radius　桡骨

rash　皮疹

ratio　The ratio of male workers to female workers in that factory is 1:3.（比例）
那家工厂的男女工人比例为1比3。

reality　Is it a reality or merely my imagination?（现实，真实存在）
那是现实还是只是我的想象而已?

repetition　Perhaps you can deepen your impression through repetition.（重复）
或许你可以通过重复来加深印象。

reproductive system　生殖系统

resistance　The so-called air resistance is a force that can slow down a moving object.（阻力，抗力）
所谓的空气阻力是一种能使运动物体减速的力。

resolve　The difficulties on the yoga path strengthened her resolve.（决心，坚定的信念）
瑜伽路上的重重困难坚定了她的决心。

respiration　Pranayama can help decrease respiration rate.（呼吸）
调息法能够帮助降低呼吸频率。

respiratory ailment　呼吸系统疾病

◆ The senses are like a mirror. Turning outward, they reflect the outside; turning inward, they reflect the pure light.

respiratory system 呼吸系统

Restorative Yoga 复元瑜伽

result As a result, they were all late for work.（结果）

结果，他们全都上班迟到了。

rheumatism 风湿

rhythm Just follow your own breathing rhythm.（节奏）

跟着自己的呼吸节奏来。

rib 肋骨

ribcage 胸腔，胸廓

rickets 佝偻病

right A yoga teacher sat on my right.（右边）

一位瑜伽老师坐在我右边。

ring finger 无名指

rope 墙绳

rose She got a bunch of roses as a gift.（玫瑰花）

她收到一束玫瑰花作为礼物。

round To quickly calm down, you may try several rounds of belly breathing.（轮次，回合）

要快速平静下来，你可以尝试几组腹式呼吸。

S

sacrum 骶骨

salutation We usually practise Sun Salutation at dawn and Moon Salutation at dusk.（致意，致意动作）

我们通常在黎明时练习拜日式，在黄昏时练习拜月式。

◆感官就像一面镜子。转向外界，它们反映外部；转向内在，它们反映出纯净的光。

sand　I enjoy the feeling of running along the sand beach.（沙子）

　　　　我享受沿着沙滩跑步的感觉。

sandbag　瑜伽沙袋

scapula　肩胛骨

scenario　In this scenario, what would you do if you were me?（情境，场景）

　　　　在这种情境下，如果你是我，你会怎么做?

sciatica　坐骨神经痛

scoliosis　脊柱侧凸，脊柱侧弯

second　Relax a few seconds before you move on to the next pose.（秒）

　　　　进行下一个体式之前先休息几秒钟。

seed　Sow the seed in a big flower pot.

　　　　把种子种在一个大花盆里。

sensation　Corpse pose can give you a very relaxing sensation.（感觉）

　　　　挺尸式可以给你一种非常放松的感觉。

shin　胫，胫骨

shinbone　胫骨

shoulder　肩膀

shoulder and neck problems　肩颈问题

shoulder blade　肩胛骨

side　Lie on your right side.

　　　　右侧卧。

silence　The whole room is in total silence.（沉默，寂静）

　　　　整个房间处于一片寂静之中。

◆ We shouldn't go to extremes but should have limitations.

sitting bone   Ground your sitting bones evenly on the floor. （坐骨）
让你的坐骨均匀落地。

skeletal system   骨骼系统

skeleton   骨骼，骨架

skull   颅骨

sky   There are so many stars in the sky. （天空）
天空中有好多星星。

slipped disc   椎间盘突出

small intestine   小肠

smoke   It smells like smoke. （烟）
闻起来像是烟的味道。

socket   Eye sockets are the places where your eyeballs normally are.
（窝、穴）
眼窝是眼球在正常情况下所在的位置。

sole   脚底

soreness   You can gently massage your calves to reduce soreness after
meditation. （疼痛、酸痛）
冥想过后你可以轻柔地按摩小腿肚以减轻酸痛。

space   Fold the blankets so they won't take so much space. （空间）
把毯子折叠起来就不会占太多空间了。

spaciousness   A high ceiling gives a feeling of spaciousness. （宽敞，
宽广）
天花板高会给人一种宽敞的感觉。

spinal column   脊柱

spine   脊柱

◆我们不应当走极端而应该有所限制。

spine injury　脊柱损伤

spleen　脾

stability　Balancing poses can improve your stability.（稳定，稳定性）
平衡体式能够提升你的稳定性。

staff　In Staff pose, you should straighten your legs in front.（拐杖，棍棒）
在手杖式中，你应当伸直双腿向前。

star　You cannot see stars on raining days.（星星）
雨天你是不会看到星星的。

starting position　起始姿势，开始位置

statement　Is this statement true or false?（表述，表达）
这种说法对还是错?

step　The next step is to lift your legs off the floor.（步，步骤）
下一步是将你的双腿抬离地板。

sternum　胸骨

stiffness　Stiffness in the back can be effectively removed through regular yoga practice.（僵硬）
通过规律性的瑜伽练习能够有效消除背部僵硬感。

stomach　胃

stomachache　胃痛，腹痛

strain　Press your forearms on the floor to take some of the strain off your wrists.（压力）
将你的小臂压向地板，以减轻手腕上的一些压力。

stream　I remember there was a stream in that woods.（溪流）
我记得那片树林里有条小溪。

◆ If you are free from your own mind and senses, nothing can bind you; then you are really free.

stress　Many people don't know how to deal with the stress in life.
（压力，紧张）

许多人不知道如何应对生活中的压力。

stretch　Bend forward and feel the stretch in your lower back.〔（四
肢或身体的）舒展，伸展〕

前屈，感受下背部的舒展。

stroke　中风

sun　The whole city is bathed in the morning sun.（太阳）

整座城市都沐浴在清晨的阳光里。

support　Put a folded blanket under your head for support.（支撑，
支撑物）

在头部下方垫一块折叠的毯子用来支撑。

surroundings　She easily adapted to the new surroundings.（环境）

她很容易地适应了新环境。

sympathetic nervous system　交感神经系统

symptom　Do you have any other symptoms?（症状）

你还有其他症状吗？

system　系统

T

tailbone　尾骨，尾椎

technique　This breathing technique is very easy to learn.（技巧，方法）

这种呼吸方法学起来很容易。

temple　太阳穴

◆如果你能从自己的思想和感官中解脱出来，就没有什么能束缚住你；
那你就真的自由了。

tension　Laughing can help release tension and stress.（紧张）

大笑能够帮助释放紧张与压力。

the back of the hand　手背

the back of the head　脑后，后脑勺

the crown of the head　头顶

the heel of the hand　掌根

the length of time　Hold for the same length of time on your right side.

（持续时间，时长）

右侧保持同样长的时间。

the outside of the foot　脚外侧

the top of the foot　脚背

thigh　大腿

thoracic vertebrae　胸椎

thought　She felt excited at the thought of attending yoga class after work.（想法）

一想到下班后去上瑜伽课她就感到兴奋。

throat　喉咙

thumb　大拇指

thyroid gland　甲状腺

tibia　胫骨

tightness　This patient has the symptoms of chest tightness and shortness of breath.（紧绷，不适）

这位患者的症状是胸闷气短。

time　When was the last time you attended yoga class?（次，回）

你上次上瑜伽课是什么时候?

◆ If we have that control (of senses), we can do whatever we want, find peace and joy within and share the same with all humanity.

tiredness　The typical symptoms of this disease include headache, tiredness and dizziness.（疲惫，疲倦）

这种疾病的典型症状包括头痛、疲劳和头晕。

toe　脚趾

toenail　脚指甲

tongue　舌头

tooth　牙齿（复数teeth）

top　I would like to have a cup of coffee with cream on top.（表面，上面）

我想来一杯上面带奶油的咖啡。

torso　躯干

total hip replacement　全髋关节置换手术

traction　The force of traction was reduced to a minimal level.（牵引，拉力）

牵引力降到了最低水平。

trapezius　斜方肌

tree　I am good at doing Tree pose.

我擅长做树式。

triangle　Your body parts form several triangles in this pose.〔三角（形）〕

在这个体式中，你的身体部位形成了几个三角形。

triceps　三头肌

trochanteric bursitis　大粗隆滑囊炎

trunk　Exhale, turn your shoulders and trunk to the right.〔（人体的）躯干〕

呼气，肩膀和躯干转动向右。

◆如果我们能控制（感官），我们就能做任何我们想做的事，找到内心的平和与喜悦，并同全人类分享。

U

ulna　尺骨

upper arm　大臂

urinary system　泌尿系统

urinary system disorder　泌尿系统紊乱

use　Use a yoga block to help you sit upright.（使用）

使用瑜伽砖帮你坐直。

V

vertebra　椎骨（复数vertebrae或vertebras）

viscera　These poses can help tone your abdominal viscera.（内脏，脏腑）

这些体式能够帮助调理你的腹部脏器。

W

waist　腰

wall　You can also try this pose with the wall as your prop.（墙）

你也可以用墙作为辅具尝试这个体式。

warrior　Warrior pose III is much more difficult than Warrior pose I.（战士，勇士）

战士三式比战士一式难多了。

way　Only in this way can we obtain more from yoga practice.（练习）

只有这样，我们才能从瑜伽练习中收获更多。

weak heart　心脏衰弱

◆ Concentration is the beginning of meditation; meditation is the culmination of concentration.

weight Many people start practising yoga because they want to lose weight.（重量）

许多人因为想减肥而开始练习瑜伽。

Shift your weight forward.（重心）

将你的身体重心前移。

width The width between two feet is about 1.5 metres.

双脚之间的距离约为1.5米。

wind I can't eat beans — they give me wind.（胃气，肠气）

我不能吃豆子，吃了肚子就胀气。(p.2304)

The wind was so strong last night.（风）

昨晚风很大。

wisdom That work requires great patience and wisdom.（智慧）

那项工作需要极大的耐心与智慧。

witness Be a witness to your mental activities in meditation.（目击者）

在冥想中做你心理活动的目击者。

woman That woman is pregnant.（妇女，女性）

那个女人怀孕了。

worry Yoga practice can help free you from the worries in the outside world.〔担心，让人发愁的事（或人）〕

瑜伽练习能够帮助你从外界的烦忧中解脱出来。

wrist 手腕

Y

yoga ball 瑜伽球

yoga block 瑜伽砖

◆专注是冥想的起点；冥想是专注的顶点。

yoga bolster 瑜伽枕

yoga mat 瑜伽垫

yoga strap 瑜伽伸展带

Yoga Therapy 瑜伽理疗

yoga wheel 瑜伽轮

Yin Yoga 阴瑜伽

◆ This very practice itself is called concentration: the mind running, your bringing it back; its running, your bringing it back. You are taming a monkey.

Verbs（动词）

A

activate　Plank pose can help activate your core muscles.（刺激，激活）
平板支撑能够帮助激活你的核心肌肉。

adjust　Adjust the position of your head.（调整，调节）
调整你头部的位置。

affirm　The yoga studio owner affirmed that no one would lose their job.（肯定）
这家瑜伽馆的老板肯定没有人会失业。

align　Align your right knee with the second toe of your right foot.（对齐，对准）
你的右膝与右脚的第二根脚趾对齐。

alleviate　Regular practice of yoga can help alleviate your menstrual discomfort.（减轻，缓和，缓解）
规律性练习瑜伽能够帮助你缓解经期不适。

analyze　She analyzed the cause and effect of this event.（分析）
她分析了这件事的前因后果。

angle　She angled her chair so that she could sit and watch the cat.
〔斜移，使成角度转向（或倾斜）〕
她斜移了椅子，以便坐着观察猫。

anchor　Make sure the tripod is securely anchored.（使固定）
确保把三脚架固定好。

◆这种练习本身就叫作专注：思想跑开，你把它带回来；它跑开，你把它带回来。你在驯服一只猴子。

arch   The cat arched its back and was ready to jump.（使弯成弓形）
猫弓起背，准备起跳。

arise   If you do not take care of your body, health problems will arise
sooner or later.（出现，上升）
如果你不照顾好自己的身体，健康问题迟早会出现。

arouse   This scene arouses a feeling that I had long time ago.（唤醒，
引起）
这一情景唤起了我很久之前有过的一种感觉。

attempt   Attempt the impossible and you will be amazed at your own
potential.（试图，尝试）
尝试不可能的事情，你会为自己的潜力感到惊讶。

avoid   People with heart failure should avoid this pose.（避免，避开）
心衰患者应避免这个体式。

B

balance   Sometimes it's hard to balance income and expenses.（使平衡）
有时很难做到收支平衡。

become   He became confused when the teacher stopped her
demonstration.（变得）
当老师停止示范时，他就开始犯糊涂了。

begin   Now, let's begin!（开始）
现在我们开始吧！

bend   I find it really hard to bend backward.（弯曲，折弯）
我发现后弯非常难。

◆ Time has no meaning in meditation, and space is also lost.

break He broke the silence and asked whether they could start the practice right now.〔打破（沉默），打断（连续性）〕
他打破沉默，问他们是否可以立刻开始练习。

breathe Deeply breathe in and slowly breathe out.（呼吸）
深深地吸气，缓缓地呼气。

bring Bring your hands behind your back.〔使朝（某方向或按某方式）移动〕
双手来到体后。

broaden The local government planned to broaden out the river.（使扩大，使变宽）
当地政府计划加宽这条河。

C

calm Calm down! This is not the end of the world.（使平静，使镇定）
冷静一下！这又不是世界末日。

catch Catch your right wrist with your left hand.（抓住，握住）
用你的左手抓住右手手腕。

centre He decided to centre his life on yoga career.（把……放在中心处）
他决定以瑜伽事业作为生活的中心。

check Please check that you lock all the windows before you leave.（查看，核实，确保）
在你离开前，请确保关上了所有窗户。

chirp I can hear sparrows chirping in the garden.（虫鸣，鸟叫）
我能听见麻雀在花园里叽叽喳喳地叫。

◆时间在冥想中没有意义，空间也失去了意义。

clasp They ran to each other and clasped hands.（紧抱，扣紧）
她们跑向对方，紧握双手。

cleanse You have to cleanse the wound before you bandage it.（净
化，使清洁）
包扎之前你得先清理一下伤口。

close Gently close your eyes and observe your breath.（关闭，闭合）
轻柔地闭合双眼，观察你的呼吸。

concave Feel your spinal column drop vertebra by vertebra starting
from your tailbone when you try to concave your back.（使
变凹形）
当你凹背时，感受脊柱从尾骨开始一节一节地向下降。

continue They decided to stay and continue practising after class.
（继续）
他们决定下课后留下来继续练习。

contract Contract your buttock muscles and press both feet into the
floor.〔（使）收缩，缩小〕
收紧臀部肌肉，双脚压向地板。

control We must learn to control our temper.（控制，管理）
我们必须学会控制自己的脾气。

correct Yoga practice can help correct your posture.（纠正，修正）
瑜伽练习能够帮你矫正身姿。

cough He coughed to attract my attention.（咳嗽）
他咳嗽几声以引起我的注意。

count He was counting the stars in the dark blue sky when I saw him.
（数数）

◆ Even the body is forgotten in real meditation... I mean, the mind transcends body consciousness.

我看见他的时候，他正在数着深蓝天空中的星星。

create Please turn off your cellphone to create a peaceful and quiet environment for yoga practice.（创造）

请关闭手机，为瑜伽练习创造一个平和安静的环境。

cross Cross your forearms and rest your hands on the shoulders.（交叉，使相交）

小臂交叉，手放在你的肩膀上。

cultivate You can cultivate patience by practising calligraphy.（培养）

你可以通过练习书法培养耐心。

curve Straighten your arms at first and then curve your body sideways.（弯，使弯曲）

先伸直手臂然后再侧向曲体。

cushion My fall was cushioned by the deep snow.（软垫，坐垫）

积雪很厚，我跌得不重。(p.492)

D

dance May I have the honor to dance with you?（跳舞）

能否有幸与你共舞?

deepen You can read this book to deepen your understanding of yoga.（使变深，加深）

你可以阅读这本书以深化对瑜伽的理解。

descend The plan began to descend.（下降）

飞机开始降落。(p.539)

desire Fight for whatever you desire.（想要，渴望得到）

为你想要的一切而奋斗。

◆在真正的冥想中，甚至连身体都被遗忘了……我的意思是，思想超越了身体意识。

develop   It usually takes a few weeks to develop a habit. （养成）

通常需要几周时间养成一个习惯。

direct   The machine directs a powerful beam at the affected part of the body. （指向）

这种机器将很强的射线对准身体感染部位。(p.560)

distribute   See that your body weight is evenly distributed on your sitting bones. （使散开，使分布，分散）

确保你的身体重量均匀地分布在坐骨上。

do   You have to find a qualified teacher to teach you how to do yoga.

〔做，干（某事）〕

你得找一位合格的老师教你如何练瑜伽。

drape   His arm was draped casually around her shoulders. （搭在，垂下）

他随意地将手臂搭在她的肩膀上。

draw   Draw your chin towards your collarbone. （拉，牵引）

将你的下巴拉向锁骨。

drop   He let his head drop. 〔（身体部位无力地）垂下，使落下〕

他垂下头。

E

elongate   As you breathe in, elongate your spine vertebra by vertebra.

（拉长，使延长）

随着吸气，一节一节地拉长你的脊柱。

empty   Would you please help me empty the trash can in the corner?

（倒空，使成为空的）

你能帮我倒一下角落里的垃圾桶吗？

◆ Liberation is not something you experience when you die. While living, you should be liberated. Jivana-mukta: mukta means liberated, jivana, while living.

end This novel ends in tragedy.（结束，终止）

这本小说以悲剧结尾。

engage I couldn't get through — the line's engaged.（使用，占用）

我打不通电话——线路忙。(p.661)

enjoy Life is short and we should learn to enjoy our life.（享受，享受……的乐趣）

人生短暂，我们应该学会享受生活。

evoke That song evoked memories of my campus life.（引起，唤起）

那首歌唤起了我对校园生活的记忆。

exercise I exercise twice a week.（锻炼，练习）

我一周锻炼两次。

exhale Hold your breath for a few seconds and then exhale.（呼气）

屏息几秒钟然后呼气。

expand You can silently observe your abdomen expand and contract.（扩张，膨胀）

你可以静静地观察你的腹部扩张和收缩。

experience I experienced a moment of anxiety when I heard the bad news.（体验，感受）

当我听到这个坏消息时感到一阵焦虑。

explore She explored the sand with her toes.〔（用手或身体某部位）探查，探索〕

她用脚趾感觉沙的情况。(p.703)

express Honestly, I don't know how to express my feelings and emotions.（表达）

实话说，我不知道如何表达自己的感受和情绪。

◆解脱不是你死后所体验到的。在你活着的时候，就应该得到解脱。Jivana-mukta: mukta的意思是解脱，jivana，在活着的时候。

extend As you inhale, extend your spine vertebra by vertebra.（延伸，伸展）

随着吸气，一节一节地延展你的脊柱。

F

face You can face forward if you feel dizzy looking upward.（面向，朝向）

如果向上看感到头晕，可以面向前方。

fall He accidentally fell from his horse.（落下）

他意外地从马上坠落。

feel Stop the practice when you feel tired or uncomfortable.（感到）

当你感到疲累或不适时，停止练习。

finish I will attend tonight's yoga class when I finish my work.（结束，完成）

工作结束后我会去上今晚的瑜伽课。

flatten He flattened the yoga mat on the floor.（使变平，使平坦）

他把瑜伽垫铺平在地板上。

flex Remember to flex your arms and legs before physical exercise.〔屈伸（肌肉或身体的某部分）〕

记得在体育锻炼之前活动一下双臂和双腿。

float A fallen leaf is floating on the water.（漂浮，漂动）

一片落叶漂浮在水面上。

flow Feel the fresh air flow smoothly into your body.〔（液体、气体或电）流动〕

感受新鲜的空气顺畅地流进你的身体。

◆ Opposites meet; extremes look alike.

follow　He has no other choice but to follow the order.（跟随）

　　　　他别无选择，只能服从命令。

force　You should not force yourself to do the final pose.（强迫，强加）

　　　　你不应该强迫自己去做终极体式。

form　Your separated legs together with the mat can form a triangle.
（形成，构成）

　　　　分开的双腿和瑜伽垫能够形成一个三角形。

G

gaze　He gazed at himself in the mirror.（凝视，注视）

　　　　他凝视着镜子里的自己。

get　It's getting warmer and warmer.（变得）

　　　　天气越来越暖和了。

give　The teacher can give a gentle push from the back.（与名词连用
描述某一动作，意义与该名词相应的动词相同）

　　　　老师可以从后面轻轻推一下。

grasp　Grasp the long end of the yoga strap with your hands.（抓牢，
握紧）

　　　　双手抓住瑜伽伸展带的长端。

grip　He griped the yoga strap.（紧握，抓住）

　　　　他紧紧抓住瑜伽伸展带。

ground　Ground your palms and feet.（使接触地面）

　　　　手掌与双脚落地。

　　◆对立相逢；极端相像。

H

happen   I have no idea what will happen in the next few days.（发生）
我不知道接下来的几天会发生什么。

have   He sat there and had his eyes closed.〔使处于（某状态）〕
他坐在那里，闭着眼睛。

help   A qualified teacher knows how to help his or her students.（帮助）
一名合格的老师知道如何帮助自己的学生。

hinge   Exhale, hinge forward from your hips and put your hands on the floor.（给……装铰链）
呼气，以髋部为折点向前，手放在地板上。

hold   Hold this pose for 5 breaths.〔使保持（在某位置）〕
在这个体式保持5个呼吸。

Could you please hold this book for me?（拿着，抓住）
你能帮我拿一下这本书吗?

hook   He was terrified because an arm hooked around his neck all of a sudden.（钩住）
他吓了一跳，因为有一只胳膊突然勾住了他的脖子。

hug   It's okay if you wear figure-hugging yoga clothes.〔缠紧，缚紧（某物，尤指人体）〕
穿紧身瑜伽服是可以的。

hunch   He hunched his shoulders and walked away.（耸肩，弓背）
他耸着肩走开了。

◆ The mind wants something. It wants to achieve this or that. What for? To be proud of itself. It develops ego.

I

imagine   Can you imagine?（想象）

你能想象到吗？

improve   This pose can improve the flexibility of your spine.（改善，提高，增进）

这个体式能增强脊柱的灵活性。

incline   That tree inclines towards the lake.（使倾斜）

那棵树向湖倾斜。

increase   You may increase the intensity of practice only when you are ready.（增加，提高）

只有当你准备好了，才能加大练习强度。

induce   These pills can induce sleep.（引起，导致）

这些药会使人昏昏欲睡。

inhale   When you inhale, feel that your belly is gradually filled with air.（吸气）

当你吸气时，感受腹部逐渐地充满气体。

interlock   Interlock your fingers, turn your palms outward and then straighten your arms.（互锁，扣紧）

十指相扣，翻转掌心向外，然后伸直你的手臂。

J

judge   We should not judge people by their appearance.（评判，评价）

我们不应当以貌取人。

◆头脑想得到一些东西。它想要实现这个或那个。对什么？为自己而骄傲。这样会助长自我。

join   There are two closed links that can join the two ends of the strap.（连接，结合）

有两个闭口环可以将伸展带的两端连在一起。

jump   Inhale and jump back to the starting position.（跳跃）

吸气，跳回到起始位置。

K

keep   Keep your feet together.（保持）

保持你的双脚并拢在一起。

kneel   Kneel on the floor.（跪下）

跪在地上。

L

lead   He led the horse to the river.（引领）

他牵着马去了河边。

lean   She leaned back in the chair.（倾斜身体）

她仰靠在椅子上。

leave   He promised that he would never leave her.（离开）

他承诺永远不会离开她。

The studio owner drove off, leaving a yoga teacher cleaning the classroom.（留下）

馆主开车走了，留下一个瑜伽老师打扫卫生。

lengthen   Lengthen your spine vertebra by vertebra.（延长，拉长）

一节一节地拉长你的脊柱。

◆ Never, never settle for these little things. Our goal is something very high. It is eternal peace, eternal joy. Don't settle for a little peace, for a little joy, for petty happiness.

let I will never let that happen again.（允许，让）

我绝不会让这样的事再次发生。

lie Take off your glasses and lie on your back.（躺，平躺）

摘掉眼镜，仰卧下来。

lift Slowly lift your head up.（举起，抬起）

慢慢地抬起你的头来。

like Do you like cooking?（像）

你喜欢做饭吗？

loop He looped the strap over his shoulder.（使成环，使绕成圈）

他把带子绕了一个圈挎在肩上。(p.1197)

loosen Massage your legs and loosen up all leg muscles.（使放松，使松弛）

按摩双腿，让双腿肌肉都放松下来。

lower Lower your feet back to the floor.（放下，降低）

双脚落回到地板上。

M

maintain Yoga practice can help you maintain a healthy heart.（维持，保持）

瑜伽练习能够帮助你保持心脏健康。

make When you teach yoga in a foreign language, try to make yourself clearly understood.（使得）

当你用外文教授瑜伽时，尽量让别人理解你的意思。

massage You can ask your partner to help massage your back.（按摩）

你可以让伙伴帮你按摩背部。

◆永远，永远不要满足于这些小事。我们的目标很高。是永恒的和平，永恒的喜悦。不要满足于一点点的和平，一点点的喜悦，一点点的幸福。

master   He soon mastered the skill of painting.（掌握，精通）
他很快掌握了绘画的技巧。

mean   I haven't seen him so far. I mean, he is late.（意味着，意思是）
到目前为止我没见到他。我的意思是，他迟到了。

measure   The teacher will measure your waistline before and after
class to see if there is any difference.（测量）
老师会在课前和课后测量你的腰围，看看是否有什么
不同。

mention   Did I ever mention that?（提及，提到）
我提到过吗？

mobilize   Certain yoga poses can help mobilize your shoulder girdle.
（使可移动）
某些瑜伽体式可以帮助你活动一下肩胛带。

move   Don't move your body in yoga nidrā.（使改变位置，移动）
在瑜伽休息术中身体不要移动。

N

need   I need your help.（需要）
我需要你的帮助。

notice   The first thing I noticed about the room was the smell.（注
意，察觉）
我首先注意到的是这屋子里的气味。(p.1363)

nourish   Yoga practice can nourish not only the body but also the soul.
（滋养）
瑜伽练习不仅可以滋养身体，也能滋养心灵。

◆ However clever we are, we can only keep the mind quiet for a little while.
Therefore, our aim is not to keep the mind peaceful but to rise above the mind and
realize the ever-peaceful Self.

O

observe He carefully observed the teacher's demonstration.（观察）

他认真地观察老师的示范。

offer The block can offer support to the upper back and help open the chest.（提供）

瑜伽砖能够支撑上背部，帮助打开胸腔。

open Could you please help me open the window?（打开）

请你帮我打开窗，好吗？

P

pass I held the door open to let her pass.（通过，经过）

我扶住打开的门，让她过去。

pause If you feel tired doing certain poses, you can pause for a moment.（暂停，停顿）

如果做某些体式感到累了，你可以暂停一会儿。

perform There are several aspects you should pay attention to if you want to perform handstand on you own.（做）

如果你想独立做手倒立的话，有几个方面你应当注意一下。

pervade The air is pervaded with the fragrance of roses.（遍及，弥漫）

空气里弥漫着玫瑰的香气。

place Place you hands on the waist.（放置）

将你的双手放在腰间。

point See that your toes point towards the ceiling.（指向，朝向）

确保你的脚趾指向天花板。

◆无论我们有多么聪明，都只能让头脑安静一小会儿。因此，我们的目标不是保持头脑平静，而是超越头脑，实现永远平静的真我。

position Position your hands beside your feet. （安置）

双手放在双脚两侧。

practise The key point is to practise regularly. （练习）

关键是要规律性练习。

prepare You have to prepare yourself for the forthcoming exams. （准备）

你得为即将到来的考试做好准备。

press Press with your palms flat on the mat. （压，按）

手掌平放在垫子上向下压。

prevent Yoga may help improve immunity and prevent certain diseases. （预防，阻止）

瑜伽可以帮助提升免疫力并预防某些疾病。

promote We should try our best to promote the public's awareness of environmental protection. （提升，促进）

我们应该尽我们所能提高公众的环保意识。

provide Our yoga studio provides tea and coffee after class. （提供）

我们的瑜伽馆课后提供茶和咖啡。

pull You pull and I'll push. （拉）

你拉，我来推。

push You can push that window open. （推）

你可以把那扇窗户推开。

R

raise Raise your legs off the mat. （提升，抬起，举起）

双腿抬起离开垫子。

◆ A changing thing cannot recognize the changes in something else, like an insane person cannot recognize the insanity of another person.

reach　He reached into his pocket and gave me a key.（伸，伸手）

他把手伸进口袋，给了我一把钥匙。

re-assume　Lower your legs down on the floor to re-assume the supine position.（再采取）

双腿落到地板上，重新采取仰卧姿势。

recline　Slowly recline on the yoga bolster.（向后倚靠）

慢慢倚靠在瑜伽抱枕上。

record　I recorded every detail in my diary.（记录，记载）

我把每个细节都记在我的日记里了。

reduce　This pose can improve blood circulation and reduce the risk of heart disease.（减少，降低）

这个体式能够促进血液循环，降低得心脏病的风险。

regularize　Practising breathing techniques can help regularize heart beat.（调整，调节）

练习呼吸技巧可以帮助调节心跳。

regulate　This air conditioner can automatically regulate the temperature in the room.（调节）

这个空调可以自动调节房间里的温度。

relax　This pose can help relax your back muscles.（放松，使松弛）

这个体式可以帮助放松背部肌肉。

release　Release your buttocks back onto the mat.（放开，松开）

臀部落回到垫子上。

Meditation is an ideal way to release tension and relax your body and mind.（使不紧张，放松）

冥想是释放紧张、放松身心的理想方式。

◆一个变化着的事物不能识别其他事物的变化，就像一个疯子不能识别另一个人的疯狂一样。

relieve   She wants to learn some yoga poses that can help relieve menstrual discomfort.（解除，减轻，缓和）

她想学习一些能够帮助缓解经期不适的瑜伽体式。

remain   Gaze forward and remain still.（保持，停留）

向前看，保持不动。

remove   This pose can help remove tiredness in your legs.（使消失）

这个体式可以消除双腿疲劳。

renew   I think it is time to renew my yoga practice.（重新开始）

我认为是时候重新开始瑜伽练习了。

repeat   Could you please repeat what you just said?（重复）

你能重复一遍你刚才说的话吗？

rest   You can rest at anytime you want.（休息）

你可以随时休息。

She rested her head on his shoulder.（使倚靠，使停放）

她的头靠在他的肩膀上。

restore   It might take a few more days to restore her to health.（恢复，使复原）

她可能还需要几天时间才能恢复健康。

retain   He struggled to retain his independence.（保持）

他努力地保持独立。

reverse   Now, you may reverse your positions.（互换，调换）

现在，你们可以互换位置了。

revitalize   Meditation is a great way to release tension and revitalize your body and mind.（使恢复生气）

冥想是释放压力、恢复身心活力的好方式。

◆ The realization doesn't stay with us for long. We should try to retain that awareness always. It will slip, but we should bring it back again and again and again. That is spiritual practice.

rise The smoke is rising from the chimney.（上升）
烟正从烟囱里升起来。

roll Roll your shoulders up, back and down.（转动）
转动你的双肩向上，向后再向下。
He rolled down a slope and broke his leg.（滚动，翻身）
他滚下斜坡摔断了腿。

rotate Rotate your shoulders back and down.（使旋转，使转动）
旋肩向后并向下。

round She rounded her lips and whistled.（使变圆）
她噘起嘴唇吹口哨。

rustle The leaves rustled in the breeze.（发出沙沙声）
树叶在微风中沙沙作响。

S

say I don't know what to say.（说）
我不知道说什么。

scan A custom officer used a detector to scan his body.（扫描）
一名海关工作人员用探测器扫描了他的身体。

sense Sense the contact of your sitting bones with the floor.（感觉，感到）
感受坐骨与地板的接触。

separate Separate your feet hip-width apart.（使分离，分开）
双脚分开与髋同宽。

shake He shook his head and refused my invitation.（摇动，晃动）
他摇摇头，拒绝了我的邀请。

◆这种领悟不会伴随我们太久。我们应该始终保持这种觉知。它会溜走，但要一次又一次地将它带回来。这就是修行。

shift   Shift the block to your right hand.（转移）

把瑜伽砖换到你的右手上。

sink   I never know a fresh egg would sink while an old one could float!
（下沉）

我从来不知道新鲜鸡蛋会下沉而陈鸡蛋可以浮起来！

sit   Sit comfortably in a chair.（坐）

舒适地坐在椅子上。

slide   Ground your sitting bones and slide your legs wide open.（滑动）

坐骨落地，双腿滑动大大地打开。

sneeze   When you sneeze, you could use a tissue to cover your nose
and mouth.（打喷嚏）

当你打喷嚏时，可以用纸巾遮盖鼻子和嘴巴。

soften   You can soften your thigh muscles through a gentle massage.
（使变柔软）

你可以通过轻柔的按摩使你的大腿肌肉变柔软。

soothe   A relaxing yoga posture can help soothe your tense and tired
muscles.（缓和，缓解）

一个放松的瑜伽体式可以帮助舒缓你紧张疲劳的肌肉。

spread   Sit on the floor and spread your legs wide apart without
overstretching.（展开，伸展）

坐在地板上，双腿大大地分开，但不要过度伸展。

That yoga teacher has more than 1 million followers spread
all over the world.（使分散，使分布）

那位瑜伽老师在世界各地有超过100万名追随者。

◆ As long as the desire to get high is there, you are not high; when you really
get high the desire fades away.

square　She squared herself to face the interviewee.（挺直身子）
　　　　她挺直身子面对面试者。

squeeze　He tried to squeeze a blanket into the closet.（挤，挤压）
　　　　他努力将一条毯子塞进壁橱里。

stand　Stand on your toes.（站立）
　　　　踮起脚尖。

start　He started to do his homework.（开始）
　　　　他开始做他的家庭作业。

stay　Stay in this pose for as long as you like.（停止，保持）
　　　　你想在这个体式中待多久就待多久。

stimulate　This prone pose can stimulate our digestive system and excretory system.（刺激，促进）
　　　　这一俯卧体式能够刺激我们的消化系统和排泄系统。

straighten　Straighten your knees and lower your feet completely on the floor.（使拉直，挺直）
　　　　双膝伸直，双脚完全落到地板上。

strain　Gently bend forward without straining.（使劲，竭力）
　　　　轻柔地前屈，不要用力。

strengthen　Practising yoga regularly can strengthen your bones and muscles.（增强，加强）
　　　　规律性地练习瑜伽可以强健骨骼与肌肉。

stretch　Stretch the front of your thighs.（伸展，拉伸）
　　　　拉伸大腿前侧。

support　Support your student's head with both hands.（支撑，支撑物）
　　　　用双手托住学生的头.

◆只要寻求兴奋的欲望存在，那你就没兴奋；当你真正兴奋的时候，这种欲望就会消失。

switch　Do you mind switching seats with me?（对调，改变方向等）

你介意和我换一下座位吗?

swivel　He swiveled around to look at her.（转身，转动）

他转过身来看着她。

T

take　Take the knees towards the chest.（引领）

双膝引领向胸部。

He stood by the window and took a deep breath.（与名词连用，表示举动、动作等）

他站在窗边，深深地吸了一口气。

It took me 2 years to finish writing this book.（花费，耗费时间）

写完这本书花了我两年时间。

throw　He threw back his head and roared with laughter.〔猛动（身体或身体部位），仰起（头）〕

他猛地仰起头哈哈大笑起来。(p.2108)

tighten　Stand still and tighten your thigh muscles.（收紧，使变紧）

站立不动，收紧你的大腿肌肉。

tone　These poses can tone your spine.（使强健，使健壮）

这些体式可以强健脊柱。

touch　May I touch your body?（接触，触碰）

我可以触碰你的身体吗?（注：辅助会员之前建议征求对方同意）

◆ The fulfillment of this desire and becoming desireless happen simultaneously.

tuck   Try tucking your shoulder blades in to open your chest a little bit more.（卷起，收拢）

试着向内收你的肩胛骨，让胸腔打开得多一点。

turn   Turn your head to face the front if you feel dizzy looking upward.（转动，转向）

如果你向上看感到头晕，那就转动头部面朝前方。

twist   He twisted his head around to look at her.〔扭转，转动（身体部位）〕

他扭过头去看她。(p.2179)

U

uncross   To come out of Eagle pose, you have to uncross your arms and legs.〔使（原交叉的腿等）还原，使不交叉〕

要退出鹰式，你得解开交叉的双臂和双腿。

use   You can use an eye pillow to cover your eyes.（使用）

你可以使用眼枕盖住你的眼睛。

V

visualize   I can't visualize what I would look like when I reach 70 or 80.（想象，设想）

我想象不出自己到了70或80岁会是什么样子。

W

walk   We walked side by side in silence.（走，走过）

我们并肩而行，一语不发。

◆欲望的满足和欲望的消失同时发生。

wander   Open your eyes when you notice your thoughts wander.（游荡，心不在焉）

当你觉察自己的思绪游离时，睁开眼睛。

want   What do you want, tea or coffee?（想要）

你想要什么，茶还是咖啡？

watch   First of all, let's watch how the teacher does it.（观察）

首先，让我们看看老师是怎么做的。

wedge   Her foot was wedged between the rocks.〔将……挤入（或塞进，插入）〕

她的脚卡在岩石之间。

widen   They may have to widen the road to cope with the increase in traffic.（变宽，扩大）

他们可能得拓宽这条道路以适应车辆的增多。

wiggle   He removed his shoes and wiggled his toes.（使扭动，摆动）

他脱掉鞋子，扭动着脚趾。（p.2301）

will   Call it what you will.（愿意，想要）

你愿意怎么称呼它就怎么称呼它。

withhold   I find it really hard to withhold from tears when hearing sad stories.（保留，抑制）

我发现很难在听到悲伤的故事后忍住眼泪。

wrap   To deepen the stretch, you can wrap a strap around your right foot and pull up.（缠绕）

要深入拉伸，你可以将伸展带缠在右脚上向上拉起。

◆ The proof of the pudding is in eating. Lick a little and see how it tastes. If it tastes good, eat a little more. It's an important point.

Prepositions（介词）

A

above　Raise your arms up above your head.（在……之上，高于）
双臂向上举过头顶。

across　It's too tight across the back.〔在（身体某部位）上〕
背部太紧。(p.17)

against　Place your elbows against the inner sides of your knees.（倚
靠，紧靠）
将你的手肘抵在双膝内侧。

along　You may look along the shelves for the book you need.（沿
着，顺着）
你可以沿着书架寻找你要的书。

alongside　Extend your arms alongside the body.（在……旁边）
让你的手臂沿身体两侧伸展。

around　Stretch the muscles around your waist.（围绕）
拉伸腰部周围的肌肉。

as　Props can work as your partner to help you deepen the poses.（作
为，当作）
辅具可以充当你的伙伴，帮助你深入体式。

at　When you practise yoga, focus on yourself and do not look at
other people.（朝，向）
当你练习瑜伽时，关注自己，不要看别人。

◆布丁怎么样，吃了才知道。稍微舔一下，看看味道如何。如果味道
好，就多吃一点。这一点很重要。

You can practise yoga at home if you can't find a good yoga studio.〔在（某处）〕

如果你找不到好的瑜伽馆的话，也可以在家练习瑜伽。

Stand upright and hold the block at arm's length.（从相隔……远的地方）

站直，拿着瑜伽砖保持一臂之远。

B

before Remember to turn off all the lights before going to bed.（在……之前）

记得睡觉前把所有的灯都关掉。

behind You could put a cushion behind your back for support.（在……后面）

你可以在背后放一个靠垫用来支撑。

below Slide your right hand along the side of your body and see if it can go below your knee.（在……下面，低于）

右手沿着身体一侧向下滑动，看它能否到膝盖以下。

beneath The boat sank beneath the waves.（在……之下）

小船被大浪吞没了。

beside The shoe rack is put beside the entrance.（在……旁边）

鞋架放在入口旁边。

between You can rest for a few seconds between two poses.（在……之间）

你可以在两个体式之间休息几秒钟。

◆ In reality, only a snake knows a snake; only a saint knows a saint.

beyond   My interests extend beyond yoga to language learning and singing.（超过，越过）

我的兴趣不仅限于瑜伽，还有语言学习和唱歌。

by   Open your chest by drawing your shoulder blades towards each other.（通过，由）

通过让肩胛骨相互靠拢来打开胸腔。

D

during   Please do not use your cellphone during the practice.（在……期间）

练习期间请不要使用手机。

F

for   You have to practise yoga for a period of time to truly experience the changes in your body and mind.（表示一段时间）

你得在练习瑜伽一段时间后才能真正体会到自己身心的改变。

What can I do for you?（以帮助，为了）

我能为您做些什么？

from   He likes neither reading nor physical activities from the very beginning.（从，从……开始）

他从一开始就既不喜欢读书也不喜欢体育活动。

I choose that yoga studio simply because it is only 1 kilometre from my home.（表示两地的距离）

我选择那家瑜伽馆不过是因为它离我家只有一公里。

◆在现实中，只有蛇了解蛇；只有圣人才了解圣人。

I

in Sit in Daṇḍāsana.（以……方式）

手杖式坐立。

Do you have a pain in your back?〔在（某范围或空间内的）某一处〕

你背部疼吗?

Many people find it hard to maintain balance in Tree pose.（在……中）

许多人感到很难在树式中保持平衡。

into Step your right foot back into Downward-facing Dog pose.（进入）

右脚后撤进入下犬式。

L

like He works like a machine.（像）

他像机器一样工作。

N

near You can put your yoga mat there, near the wall.（靠近，临近）

你可以把你的瑜伽垫放在那边，靠近墙的地方。

O

off It's extremely dangerous to get on or off the train when the door is closing.（离开）

当车门正在关闭时，上下火车是极其危险的。

◆ In one sense, you are the witness; in another, you are the actor. It depends on where you put yourself.

on   Stand on your yoga mat.（在……上）

站在瑜伽垫上。

He is hard on his kids.（与某些名词连用，表示影响到）

他对自己的孩子很严厉。(p.1390)

On an inhalation, lift your head up towards the ceiling.（在……的时候）

随着吸气，抬头向上朝向天花板。

Stand on your right foot.（由……支撑着）

右脚单腿站立。

onto   I couldn't believe he should have fallen onto his knees on a flat road!（在……上）

我不敢相信他竟然在平路上跌倒了！

outside   If you need to make a phone call, please do it outside the classroom.（在……外面）

如果你需要打电话，请到教室外面打。

over   You may put a blanket over your body in Yoga Nidrā.（在……上面）

在瑜伽休息术时你可以在身上盖一条毯子。

T

than   This pose is more challenging than that one.（比）

这个体式比那个更具有挑战性。

through   You can get what you want through hard work.（通过，经由）

你可以通过努力得到你想要的东西。

◆在某种意义上，你是目击者；从另一种意义上来说，你是行动者。这取决于你把自己放在什么位置上。

Go through this gate and you will see that the yoga studio is just on your right.（穿过）

穿过这道大门，你会看到瑜伽馆就在你的右边。

throughout He practised yoga daily throughout the year.（自始至终，贯穿）

他一整年每天都练习瑜伽。

to The teacher will come to help you in yoga class.（为了给，以提供）

老师在瑜伽课上会帮你的。

Her weight dropped to 50 pounds.〔（范围或时间的结尾或界限）到，至〕

她的体重降到了50磅。

Come to the top end of your yoga mat.（到达某处）

来到你垫子的顶端。

toward Bring your knees toward your chest.（朝向）

将双膝拉向胸部。

U

under You may place a folded blanket under your right knee.（在下面）

你可以在右膝下方放一条折叠的毯子。

underneath Your cellphone is left underneath the yoga mat.（在……底下）

你的手机落在瑜伽垫下面了。

◆ Either act and be responsible, or allow the mind and body to act and be a witness, totally free.

W

with You can try this pose with your eyes closed.（伴随）

你可以尝试闭眼做这个体式。

People with high blood pressure should be careful with this pose.（有）

有高血压的人应当谨慎做这个体式。

You may cover your body with a thin blanket.（用，使用）

你可以用薄毯子盖住身体。

without He has been working for 10 days without a break.（没有，不带）

他连续工作了10天没有休息。

Adjectives & Adverbs（形容词 & 副词）

A

abdominal　If you want to strengthen your abdominal muscles, you could try plank pose.（腹部的）

如果你想增强腹肌，可以试试平板支撑。

about　About 3 people in this class can do headstand.（大约，将近）

这个班里大约有3个人能做头倒立。

above　If you want to know more about this course, please call the above number.（在……之上，高于）

关于这个课程如果你想了解更多，请拨打上面这个电话。

abundant　We can continuously provide abundant teaching resources.（充裕的，丰富的）

我们能够持续不断地提供丰富的教学资源。

active　Bats are active only at night.（活跃的，起作用的）

蝙蝠仅在夜间活动。

actively　He has been actively solving these problems.（主动地，积极地）

他一直在积极地解决这些问题。

acute　It's an acute disease.（急性的）

它是一种急性病。

◆ Karma Yoga — selfless service without personal expectation — is done by the mind.

adjoining This backward bending pose can strengthen the lower back and other adjoining parts of the body.（邻近的，毗邻的）

这一后弯体式能够强健下背部及其他相邻身体部位。

again May I try again?（再一次，又）

我可以再试一次吗？

all You might practise yoga at all times and in all places.（全部的，所有的）

你可以随时随地练习瑜伽。

almost It's almost finished.（几乎，差不多）

差不多完成了。

already The door was already open.（已经）

门已经打开了。

alternate This cake has alternate layers of fruit and chocolate.（交替的）

这个蛋糕是水果和巧克力层相间的。

apart Stand with your feet slightly apart.（相距，分开）

双脚微微分开站立。

B

back Rotate your shoulders back and down.（*adv.* 向后地）

双肩转动向后并向下。

Turn the back foot slightly in.（*adj.* 后面的）

后脚稍向内收。

backward He closed his eyes and walked backward.（向后地）

他闭上眼睛倒退着走。

◆行动瑜伽——没有个人期待的无私服务——是由心灵完成的。

bare   She likes walking indoors in bare feet.（赤裸的）

她喜欢光脚在屋里走。

beautifully   This book is beautifully printed.（漂亮地）

这本书印刷精美。

bound   We shouldn't be bound by others' values.（受约束的，被限制的）

我们不应该被他人的价值观束缚住。

bright   I remember we went out hiking on a bright spring day.（明亮的）

我记得我们在一个明媚的春日出去远足。

C

calm   Try to keep calm in case of emergency and ask for help immediately.（冷静的，平静的）

遇到紧急状况时尽量保持冷静并立即寻求帮助。

carefully   If you want to try an advanced pose, do it under the supervision of a teacher or do it very carefully in an open area.（小心地，仔细地）

如果你想尝试高级体位，在老师的监督下进行或者在开阔区域十分小心地尝试。

clear   — Are you clear now?（清楚的）

——你现在清楚了吗?

— Crystal clear!

——十分清楚!

◆ The entire life is an open book, a scripture. Read it. Learn while digging a pit or chopping some wood or cooking some food. If you can't learn from your daily activities, how are you going to understand the scriptures?

clinically depressed   Those that are clinically depressed should seek a doctor's advice before practising yoga.（临床抑郁症的）

通过临床诊断得了抑郁症的人在练习瑜伽前应当征求医生的建议。

colorful   In her eyes, life is so colorful.（富有色彩的，多彩的）

在她看来，生活是多姿多彩的。

comfortable   You are advised to dress in comfortable clothes when practising meditation.（舒适的，舒服的）

建议你在练习冥想时，衣着舒适。

comfortably   Lie comfortably on the mat.（舒服地，舒适地）

舒服地躺在垫子上。

competent   Obtaining a teaching certificate doesn't mean you are a very competent teacher.（有能力的，能胜任的）

获得教师资格证书并不意味着你就是一名很有能力的教师。

complete   We were in complete agreement.（完整的，完全的）

我们意见完全一致。(p.402)

completely   I completely understand what you just said.（完全地，全然的）

我完全明白你刚才所说的话。

consciously   As a devoted yoga practitioner, she lived her life consciously.（有意识地）

作为一名虔诚的瑜伽练习者，她有意识地生活着。

◆整个人生是一本打开的书，一本经典。阅读它。在挖坑、劈柴或做饭的时候学习。如果你不能从你的日常活动中学习，你将如何理解这些经典呢？

continuous We will provide better service through continuous improvement.（连续的，连绵不断地）
我们将通过持续改进提供更好的服务。

cross-legged Sit comfortably in a cross-legged position.（盘着腿的）
舒适地盘腿坐着。

D

dark People in this village usually stay indoors when it gets dark.（黑暗的，深色的）
这个村子里的人通常天一黑就待在家里。

dark blue She has dark blue eyes and blond hair.（深蓝色的）
她有深蓝色的眼睛和金色的头发。

deep Try to keep your breathing long and deep.（深的）
尽量让你的呼吸深长。

deeply He was deeply touched by the movie.（深深地）
他被这部电影深深地打动了。

devastated He was devastated to know that his dog was poisoned.（极度悲痛的，极为不安的）
得知他的狗被毒死了，他感到伤心欲绝。

different There are actually many different schools of yoga.（不同的）
实际上有许多不同的瑜伽流派。

directly The teacher stood directly opposite to me.（直接地，正好地）
老师站在我的正对面。

down Lie down on the floor.（向下，在下面）
躺在地板上。

◆ Happiness is not to be sought outside. It can never come from outside or from inside. It can't come—because it simply is. It is always like this. Where is happiness? Everywhere.

downward   Press your palms downward.（向下）

将你的手掌向下压。

drooping   He stood there with a drooping head.（下垂的）

他低着头，站在那儿。

E

effective   Effective measures should be taken to deal with air pollution.
（有效的，起作用的）

应当采取有效措施处理空气污染。

either   You may take either road as you like.〔（两者中的）任一的〕

你想走哪条路都可以。

elevated   The injured leg should remain elevated.（抬高的）

受伤的腿应当保持抬高。

enough   She is competent enough to be your teacher.（足够地，充足地）

她有足够的能力当你的老师。

entire   He had spent his entire life teaching yoga all over the world.
（全部的，整个的）

他一生都在世界各地教授瑜伽。

equal   These two yoga mats are equal in length.（相同的，相等的）

这两张瑜伽垫长度一样。

equally   Make sure that both sides of your body are equally stretched.
（相等地，同样）

确保身体两侧得到同样的拉伸。

◆幸福是不能从外界求得的。它既不来自外部，也不来自内部。它不会来——因为幸福就是幸福。总是这样。幸福在哪里？它无处不在。

erect   Stand with your arms by your side and your head erect.（直立的，笔直的）

手放两边，昂首站立。(p.674)

especially   The weather is very hot in summer, especially in August.（尤其，特别是）

夏天天气十分炎热，尤其是八月份。

even   Press both feet with even strength.（均衡的，相等的）

双脚均匀用力向下压。

evenly   Try to breathe evenly.（均匀地，平等地）

试着均匀地呼吸。

excess   Excess food is stored as fat.（过量的，过剩的）

多余的食物作为脂肪贮存起来。(p.691)

existing   These existing problems should be solved immediately.（存在的）

现存的这些问题应当被立即解决掉。

extended   Make sure that both your arms and legs are fully extended.（延长的，扩展的）

确保你的手臂和双腿都充分地伸展。

external   You can create a favorable external environment for your yoga practice at home.（外部的）

你可以在家为自己的瑜伽练习创造一个良好的外部环境。

extreme   He walked with extreme caution.（极度的）

他极其谨慎地走着。

◆ Every personal attachment is a knot that binds you. Untie yourself. You don't have to give up anything in this world, only your attachments to them. You may possess things, but don't let them possess you.

F

far The yoga studio is not far from here.（很远地）

瑜伽馆离这里不远。

farther We watched their ship moving gradually farther away.（更远地，更进一步地）

我们望着他们的船渐渐远去。(p.729)

female He recalled that he heard a gentle female voice before he passed out.（女性的）

他回忆说，在他昏倒之前，他听到了一个轻柔的女声。

final Take it easy. Do not rush to the final pose.（最终的）

慢慢来。不要着急做到终极体式。

finally Keep practising and I'm sure you will finally make it.（最终，最后）

坚持练习，我相信你最终会成功的。

firm Keep both feet on the ground, firm and steady.（稳固，强有力的）

保持双脚落地，有力而稳定。

first Let me finish my yoga practice first.（首先）

让我先完成瑜伽练习。

fixed Gaze at a fixed point in front of your face.（固定的）

盯着眼前固定的一点。

flat Lie flat on the yoga mat and breathe deeply.（adv. 平直地）

平躺在瑜伽垫上，深呼吸。

You can get a flat stomach by practising yoga.（*adj.* 平的，平坦的）

通过练习瑜伽，你可以让腹部平坦。

◆每一个个人依附都是绑住你的结。解开自己。你不必放弃这个世界上的任何东西，只要放弃你对它们的依附。你可以拥有东西，但不要让它们掌控你。

folded Put a folded blanket under your buttocks. （折叠的）

在你的臀部下方放一条折叠的毯子。

forward Stretch both arms forward. （*adv.* 向前地）

双臂向前伸展。

Forward bending poses are really difficult for me. （*adj.* 向前的）

前屈体式对我而言真的很难。

front Shift your weight to the front leg. （前面的）

将你的身体重心转移到前腿上。

full A full-length mirror can help beginners to adjust their yoga poses. （完全的，完整的）

全身镜能够帮助初学者调整他们的瑜伽体式。

fully I fully understand your thoughts and feelings. （充分地，完全地）

我完全理解你的想法和感受。

further Could you please further explain this phenomenon with an example? （进一步地，更远地）

请你举个例子进一步解释一下这个现象可以吗？

G

gentle He spoke slowly with a gentle smile on his face. （温和的，轻柔的）

他缓缓道来，脸上挂着温柔的笑。

gently Gently open your eyes. （轻轻地，温和地）

轻柔地睁开你的眼睛。

◆ Test all your desires and actions... "Will this affect my peace?" No? Okay, let it be. But if the answer is, "My peace will be disturbed," stay away.

gone　That kind of lifestyle was gone for good.（离去的，不复存在的）

那种生活方式一去不返了。

gradually　Gradually, you can do the final pose on your own.（逐步地，渐渐地）

逐渐地，你可以独立完成终极体式。

green　Do you want green tea or black tea?（绿色的）

你想要绿茶还是红茶?

guided　No worries, you will be guided throughout the practice.（有指导的）

不用担心，全程练习都会有人指导你。

H

half　He drank half a cup of tea after class.（一半的）

他在下课后喝了半杯茶。

happily　They chatted happily with each other.（快乐地，愉快地）

他们彼此愉快地交谈着。

happy　Happy weekend!（高兴的，快乐的，幸福的）

周末愉快!

healthy　I want to live a healthy life.（健康的）

我想要过健康的生活。

heart-breaking　I guess I would never forget that heart-breaking experience.（令人心碎的）

我想我可能永远不会忘记那段令人心碎的经历。

heavy　This schoolbag is too heavy for a 6-year-old student.（沉重的）

这个书包对一个6岁学生来说太沉了。

◆考验你所有的欲望和行动……"这会影响我的平静吗？"不会？好吧，随它去。但如果答案是，"我的平静会被打扰"，离它远点。

high   This mountain is higher than that one.（高的）
这座山比那一座高。

horizontally   Stretch your arms horizontally.（水平地）
让你的双臂水平伸展。

I

immediately   You are advised not to take a shower immediately after yoga practice.（立即，直接地）
建议你不要在瑜伽练习后马上洗澡。

important   This yoga training program is very important to me.（重要的）
这个瑜伽培训项目对我而言非常重要。

in   Turn your left foot slightly in.（在里面）
左脚稍向内收。

inner   This pose can gently stretch your inner groin.（内部的）
这个体式可以轻柔地拉伸你的腹股沟内侧。

inside   It's so cold outside. Let's go inside.（在里面）
外面太冷了。咱们进去吧。

introverted   She was once a kind and introverted child.（内向的）
她曾经是一个善良且内向的孩子。

inward   Meditation is a process of turning inward.（向内的）
冥想是一个转向内在的过程。

◆ The greatest power on earth is thought-force. Before you make your thoughts powerful, first make the mind clean.

J

just　This dress is just my size.（刚好，恰好）

　　这件裙子的尺码刚好适合我。

L

last　He is always the first to come and the last to leave.（最后的）

　　他总是第一个来，最后一个走。

laterally　Bending laterally can help reduce the fat in your waist.（旁边地）

　　侧弯能够帮助减少你腰部的脂肪。

left　Now, repeat on the left side.（左边的）

　　现在，换左侧重复（练习）。

less　Nowadays people eat more but exercise less.（更少地）

　　现如今人们吃得更多但运动得更少。

light　This yoga mat is lighter than that one.（轻的，lighter更轻的）

　　这张瑜伽垫比那张更轻。

lightly　Lightly rotate your shoulders back and down.（轻轻地）

　　轻轻地旋肩向后并向下。

long　Take a long, deep breath.（长的）

　　深长地吸一口气。

lower　This sitting pose can help relax your lower back.（下方的，下面的）

　　这个坐立体式能够帮助放松你的下背部。

◆地球上最伟大的力量是思想的力量。在让你的思想变得强大之前，先让你的思想洁净。

M

mental   He is in a good mental status.（精神的，脑力的，心理上的）
他的精神状态很好。

mentally   The fact is she is likely mentally challenged.（精神上，智
力上，心理上）
事实是她可能是智力障碍者。

mild   She looked at the teacher with a look of mild confusion.（轻微的）
她略带困惑地看着老师。

more   It's more difficult to make money these days.（*adv.* 更多，此
外，更大程度地）
现在挣钱更难了。

I guess I need more time to practise this pose.（*adj.* 更多的）
我想我需要更多的时间来练习这个体式。

motionless   She was standing there as motionless as a statue when he
found her.（一动不动）
当他发现她时，她站在那里像一尊雕像一样一动
不动。

N

natural   If someone criticizes you, it's natural that you feel sad.（自然的）
如果有人批评你，你感到难过是很自然的。

naturally   Meditation can never be forced to happen. Instead, it
happens naturally.（自然地）
冥想从来不会被迫发生。相反，它是自然而然发生的。

◆ Even when you are physically doing something, your aim can be meditation.
After all, what is meditation? Focusing your entire mind on what you are doing.

necessary It's not necessary to bring your own yoga mat.（必要的，必需的）

不必自带瑜伽垫。

neutral Try to maintain a neutral spine.（中和的，不引起变化的）

试着保持脊柱位置中正。

never I swear I would never do it again!（从不，决不）

我发誓再也不这样做了！

next He will become a registered yoga teacher next month.（紧接在后的，下一个）

下个月他将成为一名注册瑜伽教师。

normal His reaction is quite normal.（正常的，标准的）

他的反应很正常。

normally Hold the pose and breathe normally.（正常地，通常地）

保持体式，正常呼吸。

O

objective He has no objective evidence to prove his innocence.（客观的）

他没有客观证据证明自己的清白。

only Only the boss can use this room.（只有）

只有老板才能使用这个房间。

opposite East and west are opposite directions.（相反的，对立的）

东和西是反方向。

◆即使你正在做一些体力上的事情，你的目标也可以是冥想。毕竟，冥想是什么？把你全部的注意力集中在你正在做的事情上。

outer　Shift your centre of gravity onto your right leg and the outer edge of your right feet.（外部的）

将你的重心转移到右腿和右脚外缘上。

outward　You should push outward to open the door.（向外）

你应该向外推才能打开门。

overhead　Raise both arms overhead.（在头顶上方）

双臂举过头顶。

P

parallel　Make your arms parallel to each other.（平行）

让你的双臂互相平行。

peaceful　Getting close to nature gives me a peaceful feeling.（和平的，平静的）

接近大自然给我一种平静的感觉。

personal　That's her personal opinion.（个人的，私人的）

那是她个人观点。

personally　Personally speaking, I prefer traditional yoga practice.（关于个人的）

就个人来说，我更喜欢传统的瑜伽练习。

previously　He told me that the yoga studio was previously owned by a young lady.（先前地）

他告诉我这家瑜伽馆先前归一位年轻女士所有。

physical　Physical exercise is good for your health.（身体的）

锻炼身体对你的健康有益。

◆ Learn to live a natural life. First be physically at ease; mental peace will automatically follow. Live in a way that makes your body light, healthy, and more supple.

physically The research has shown that physically active animals have better memories. （肉体的，身体上的）
研究表明身体活跃的动物拥有更好的记忆力。

pink She is dressed in pink sportswear. （粉红的）
她穿着粉色运动服。

pleasant The teacher's voice is really pleasant to hear. （令人愉快的）
老师的声音非常好听。

positive We should adopt a positive attitude. （积极的）
我们应该采取积极态度。

prone Lie prone on the ground. （俯卧的）
俯卧在地上。

properly Remember to check whether your back is properly supported. （恰当地，正确地）
记得检查一下你的背部是否得到了适当的支撑。

protruding Make sure that your ribs are not protruding. （突出的，伸出的）
确保你的肋骨不向外突出。

Q

quickly She walks very quickly to the door. （迅速地，快速地）
她快速走向门口。

quietly She quietly waited there with no expression on her face. （安静地，静静地）
她静静地在那里等着，脸上毫无表情。

◆学会过一种自然的生活。首先身体要放松；精神平静随之而来。以一种让你的身体轻盈、健康和更柔软的方式生活。

R

raised He tried to speak in a raised voice.（抬高的，举起的）

他努力提高嗓门讲话。

ready Are you ready for the class?（准备好）

你准备好上课了吗?

recent The yoga studio has changed a lot in recent years.（最近的，

近期的）

近几年瑜伽馆变化很大。

reclining I bought a new adjustable reclining chair.（倾斜的，向后

倚靠的）

我买了一个新的可调节式躺椅。

relatively Forward bending poses are relatively easy for me.（相

对地）

前屈体式对我而言相对简单些。

relaxed The atmosphere in the yoga studio is comfortable and relaxed.

（放松的，平静的）

瑜伽馆里的氛围是舒适放松的。

respective They are each recognized specialists in their respective

fields.（分别的）

他们在各自的领域里都被视为专家。(p.1699)

right Raise your right hand if you have any questions.（右边的）

如果有任何问题请举右手。

◆ By nature we are at ease and in peace. However, due to negligence or efforts aimed at satisfying selfish desires of the senses, we disturb that ease and peace.

S

same   These two yoga blocks are of the same brand.（相同的）

这两块瑜伽砖是同一品牌的。

seated   Please remain seated until the aircraft has come to a halt.（就座的，坐下的）

飞机停好以前，请坐着别动。

serious   Obesity has become a serious health problem.（严重的）

肥胖已经成为一个严重的健康问题。

several   Hold this pose for several minutes.（几个的）

在这个体式中保持几分钟。

short   He sent me a short message.（简短的）

他给我发了条短信。

sideways   He fell sideways from the wall.（向侧面的，向一旁的）

他从墙上侧着摔下来了。

silently   Silently listen to the teacher's instructions.（静静地，默默地）

静静地听老师的口令。

simple   Many people practise yoga for the simple reason that they want to lose weight.（纯粹的，完全的）

许多人之所以练习瑜伽，纯粹是因为他们想减肥。

simultaneously   Yoga practice can improve your flexibility and strength simultaneously.（同时地）

瑜伽练习能够同步提升你的灵活性和力量。

◆我们生性安逸平和。然而，由于我们的粗心大意或为满足感官的自私欲望而耗费心力，我们破坏了这种安逸与平和。

single　I didn't receive a single message from her.〔一个的（用于强调）〕

　　　　我没收到她的任何消息。

slightly　Stand with your feet apart, slightly wider than your hips.（稍微地，轻微地）

　　　　站立时，双脚打开略宽于髋。

slow　The progress is slow but steady.（慢的）

　　　　进展缓慢但很稳定。

slowly　Slowly open your eyes and feel the peace within.（缓慢地，慢慢地）

　　　　慢慢睁开你的眼睛，感受内心的平静。

small　The teacher noticed several small errors in his teaching plan.（不重要的，些微的）

　　　　老师注意到他的教案里有几处小错。

smooth　That airplane made a smooth landing.（平稳的，连续而流畅的）

　　　　那架飞机平稳降落。

snow-capped　A snow-capped mountain is a mountain covered with snow at the top.（山顶被雪覆盖的）

　　　　雪山是指山顶被雪覆盖的山。

so　If you feel painful when I touch your back, please say so.〔如此（用以指代刚刚提及的事）〕

　　　　如果我碰你的背部时你感到疼痛，请直接告诉我。

　　　　I'm so glad to see you here.（如此，这么）

　　　　我很高兴在这儿见到你。

◆ We have to keep the variety and rise above it to see the unity. We need the variety, but we can enjoy the variety only if we always keep in mind the unity behind it.

soft This face cream can keep your skin soft and moisturized.（软的，柔软的）

这种面霜能让你的皮肤保持柔软湿润。

spinal Those that have spinal injuries should avoid this pose.（脊柱的）

脊椎损伤的人应当避免这个体式。

steady Keep a nice and steady breathing rhythm.（稳定的，稳固的）

保持良好稳定的呼吸节奏。

step-by-step Our Teacher Training program provides step-by-step tutorials online.（循序渐进的）

我们的教师培训项目在线提供循序渐进的教程。

still Still water runs deep.（静止的，不动的）

静水流深。

straight Keep your arms and legs straight.（*adj.* 直的，笔直的）

保持你的手臂和双腿伸直。

Look straight ahead.（*adv.* 直地，径直地）

目视前方。

strongly The wind blew strongly last night.（强有力地）

昨晚风刮得很大。

supple I'm quite supple because I practise yoga every day.（灵活的，柔软的）

我身体很柔软，因为我每天都练习瑜伽。

◆我们必须保持多样性并超越多样性看到统一。我们需要多样性，但只有我们始终记住它背后的统一才能享受多样性。

T

then   He made a good start when doing handstand, but then he fell to the ground.（然后）

他做手倒立的时候开了个好头，然而后来摔倒在地。

therefore   He's only 16 years old and therefore he is not eligible to get married.（因此）

他只有16岁，因此不具有结婚的资格。

thickly   The bread was thickly sliced.（厚厚地）

面包切得很厚。

tight   His body becomes so tight due to nervousness.（紧的，紧绷的）

由于紧张，他的身体变得十分僵紧。

tired   I feel so tired after a day's work.（疲倦的）

一天工作结束后，我感到十分疲累。

together   Now, let's practise together.（一起）

现在，我们来一起练习。

top   That book, *The Yoga Sutras of Patanjali*, is kept on the top shelf.（最高的，最上面的）

那本《帕坦伽利的瑜伽经》放在最上面的架子上。

totally   I totally agree with you.（完全地）

我完全同意你的看法。

twinkling   You could see twinkling lights when you look out of this window at night.（闪烁的）

晚上当你从这扇窗户望出去时，你会看到灯光闪烁。

◆ What fell into your mind to disturb it? Certainly nothing from outside can fall in, unless you allow something to happen to your mind.

U

unable Bend your knees if you are unable to lower your feet completely on the floor.（不能的）

如果你无法将双脚完全落到地板上，那就屈膝。

unaffected She was totally unaffected by what just happened.（不受影响的）

她完全不受刚才所发生的事情的影响。

under She took a deep breath before she went under.（在下面）

她潜下水之前深吸了一口气。

up Raise your arms up towards the ceiling.（在上面，向上）

让你的手臂上举朝向天花板。

upper This pose can strengthen your upper limbs.（上面的）

这个体式能够强健你的上肢。

upright Stand upright with your hands relaxed alongside your body.（挺直的，直立的）

站直，双手于身体两侧放松。

upward Lift your legs upward towards the ceiling.（向上地）

让你的双腿向上抬起朝向天花板。

W

weightlessly Willow catkins are floating weightlessly in the sky.（无重量地）

柳絮在空中轻盈地飘舞。

well I can well understand your worries.（很好地，充分地）

我非常理解你所担心的。

◆是什么进入你的头脑搅乱了你的思绪？当然，任何外来的东西都不能进入你的头脑，除非你允许某些事情发生在你的头脑里。

white   In yoga tradition, white color stands for purity.（白色的）

在瑜伽传统中，白色代表纯洁。

whole   She devoted her whole body and mind to yoga teaching career.（整个的，全部的）

她全身心地投入瑜伽教学事业中。

wide   She was wide awake during the process of Yoga nidrā.（充分地）

她在瑜伽休息术时保持全然地清醒。

widely   Sit in Daṇḍāsana and then widely spread your legs.（大大地，很大程度地）

手杖式坐立，然后双腿大大地分开。

within   Changes should be made from within.（在内部，在里面）

改变应该从内部开始。

◆ Nobody can always be completely happy without knowing that he or she is happiness.

Phrases（词组）

A

a cloud of   A cloud of birds flew by.（一团，一大片）
一大群鸟飞过。

a few   She asked the teacher a few questions after class.（一些，几个）
她课下问了老师几个问题。

a few more   I guess you'll need to wait a few more days.（再多几个）
我想你需要再多等几天。

align with   Make sure your front heel is aligned with the midline of
your back foot.（对齐）
确保你的前脚脚跟与后脚中线对齐。

a little   I feel a little tired.（一点儿）
我感到有点累。

a little bit more   Allow your back to descend a little bit more when
you feel ready.（再多一点儿）
当你感到准备好了，让你的背部下沉的更多
一点。

allow...to...   Please allow me to introduce myself.（允许）
请允许我做一下自我介绍。

a round of   These two yoga studios started a new round of competition.
（一轮）
这两家瑜伽馆开始了新一轮的竞争。

◆如果不知道自己就是幸福，没有人能永远完全幸福。

as...as possible   We hope to meet you as soon as possible. (尽可能……)

我们希望尽快见到您。

as far as possible   Lift your heels as far as possible. (尽可能地)

尽量抬起你的脚跟。

as far as you can   As far as you can remember, how many poses did we learn last class? (尽你所能)

据你所能想起的，上节课我们学了多少个体式?

as long as   You can finally make it as long as you stick to the end. (只要)

只要你坚持到底，你最终会成功的。

as though   I feel as though my state of mind has totally changed. (好像，仿佛)

我感觉自己的心态好像完全改变了。

at eye level   Computer screens should be at eye level. (在视线的水平高度)

计算机屏幕应该与视线齐平。

at least   I advise you to practise yoga at least twice a week. (至少)

我建议你一周至少练习两次瑜伽。

at one's own pace   If you choose online learning, you can study at your own pace. (以某人自己的节奏)

如果你选择线上学习，那么你就可以按自己的节奏来学习了。

at the beginning of   We will chant Om three times at the beginning of our today's practice. (在……的开始)

在今天的练习开始时，我们将唱三遍Om。

◆ All trouble and turmoil are blessings in disguise.

away from Stay away from computer games.（远离，离开）

远离电脑游戏。

B

balance on Some standing poses require you to balance on one leg.

〔使（在某物上）保持平衡〕

一些站立体式要求你单腿平衡站立。

be able to He is able to look after himself now.（能够）

他现在能自己照顾自己了。

be advised to Students are advised to review what they have learned

at school.（被建议）

建议学生复习在学校所学的知识。

be aware of He is fully aware of the current situation.（意识到，察

觉到）

他完全了解目前的形势。

(be) based on This sequence, based on your personal health

condition, is designed by a yoga teacher with 5 years'

teaching experience.（基于）

根据您的个人健康状况，一位有5年教学经验的瑜

伽老师设计了这个序列。

be careful (not) to I have to be careful not to catch cold these days.

〔小心（不要）〕

这些天我得小心别感冒了。

◆所有的麻烦和混乱都是伪装的祝福。

be careful with Please be careful with this pose if you have high blood pressure.（对……小心，警惕）

如果你有高血压，请小心练习这个体式。

be experienced in She is fairly experienced in teaching yoga.（在……方面有经验）

她在瑜伽教学方面相当有经验。

be familiar with She is very familiar with the surroundings here.（熟悉）

她对这里的环境非常熟悉。

be full of This space is full of love and peace.（充满）

这个空间充满了爱与和平。

(be) given by This Sanskrit name was given by my teacher in 2019.（由……给予的）

这个梵文名字是2019年由我的老师起的。

(be) parallel to Straighten your arms and make sure they are parallel to each other.（与……平行）

手臂伸直，确保双臂互相平行。

(be) rooted in This faith is deeply rooted in everyone's heart.（植根于，深植于）

这种信念深深扎根在每个人的心里。

be suitable for These yoga clothes are really suitable for you.（适合）

这些瑜伽服很适合你。

be supported by In this pose, your whole body is supported by your forearms and palms.（由……所支撑）

在这个体式中，你的整个身体是由小臂和手掌支撑。

◆ If you know the purpose of suffering—to burn up your ego—you will even rejoice in it. Suffering is a way of purification.

bear in mind　Please bear in mind that safety always comes first.（记住，牢记在心）

请记住安全永远是第一位的。

before bed　You can read a few pages before bed.（睡觉之前）

你可以睡前读几页。

begin with　Usually, yoga classes begin with mantra chanting.（以……开始，开始于……）

通常情况下，瑜伽课是以曼陀罗唱诵开始的。

between...and...　You can practise meditation between 5p.m. and 7p.m.（在……与……之间）

你可以在下午5点到7点间练习冥想。

both...and...　Both Tree pose and Mountain pose are standing poses.（两者都）

树式和山式都是站立体式。

breathe out　When you breathe out, feel your body and mind totally relaxed.（呼气）

当你呼气时，感受你的身心完全放松下来。

bring back to life　The doctor tried his best but failed to bring the patient back to life.（使重生，使复活）

医生尽了最大努力但也没能使病人起死回生。

C

carry...into...　Try not to carry your personal emotions into your work.（把……带进）

尽量不要把私人情绪带到工作中。

◆如果你知道痛苦的目的——烧掉你的自我——你甚至会因此而高兴。痛苦是一种净化的方式。

catch hold of　Catch hold of the strap with both hands.（抓住）
双手抓住伸展带。

cave in　Don't cave in your chest if you want to maintain a good posture.
（塌陷，凹进）
如果你想要保持良好的体态就不要含胸。

choose to　Whatever you say, I choose to believe you.（选择）
无论你说什么，我都选择相信你。

clear one's throat　He cleared his throat and then started his speech.
（清清嗓子）
他清了清嗓子，然后开始演讲。

close to　I want to live close to nature.（靠近，接近）
我想要接近大自然而生活。

come back　The expert predicted that everything would come back to
normal within a month.（恢复原状）
专家预测一切将在一个月内恢复正常。

come back to　Hands down and feet together to come back to the
starting position.（返回到）
双手放下，双脚并拢，回到起始位置。

come down　Come down from the hammock.（下来）
从吊床上下来。

come out of　When you are ready, you can come out of the pose.
（从……中出来）
当你准备好了，就可以退出体式了。

◆ Just as gold ore is repeatedly heated and cooled to raise its purity, all
individuals are purified by the heat of suffering.

come to She came to the yoga studio by bus.（来到，到达）

她乘坐公交来瑜伽馆。

come to an end Our winter holiday is coming to an end.（结束）

我们的寒假就要结束了。

come up To come up, rock your body back and forth and finally sit on the mat.（上来，起来）

要起来时，身体前后摆动，最后坐到垫子上。

concentrate on Concentrate on what you are doing now.（全神贯注，集中精力于）

专注于你当下正在做的事情。

coordinate with Each movement of your hands should coordinate with that of your feet.（使与……协调，配合）

手和脚的每一个动作要协调。

count numbers When you feel angry, try to count numbers to calm down.（计数，数数）

当你感到生气时，试着数数让自己平静下来。

culminate in Weeks of reports will culminate in a formal presentation in the final class.（达到顶点，以……告终）

数周的报告将会以最后一节课的正式展示而告终。

D

depend on You may perform the final pose or its variation, depending on your own condition.（取决于）

你可以根据自己的情况做终极体式或它的变体。

◆就像金矿石被反复加热和冷却以提高其纯度一样，所有人都在痛苦的灼热中得到净化。

E

each other   Practitioners can help each other in Partner Yoga.（彼此，互相）

在双人瑜伽中，练习者可以互相帮助。

embark on   Are you ready to embark on a new program?（着手做）

你准备好着手一个新项目了吗?

extend out   Extend both legs out at the same time.（伸出，伸展）

双腿同时伸出。

F

fall asleep   Don't fall asleep in meditation.（入睡，睡着）

冥想时不要睡着。

fall on   Lift up your toes and feel the weight of your body falls on the rest of your feet.（落到，落在）

脚趾抬起，感受身体重心落在双脚其他部位。

focus on   Try to focus on your breath and your feelings at the moment.（集中于，关注）

试着关注你的呼吸以及你当下的感受。

force oneself   Don't force yourself to do anything that goes against your will.（强迫自己）

不要强迫自己做任何违背自己意愿的事。

for example   For example, you may use blocks or straps to help with your practice.（举例）

举例来说，你可以使用瑜伽砖或伸展带辅助练习。

◆ Unless the body is perfectly healthy and free from all toxins and tensions, a comfortable pose is not easily obtained.

for the sake of　More and more people start to practise yoga for the sake of physical health.（为了）

越来越多的人为了身体健康而开始练习瑜伽。

free...from...　Regular yoga practice can free your body from stiffness.（摆脱）

规律的瑜伽练习可以使你的身体摆脱僵硬。

from...to...　He decided to drive from Tianjin to Qingdao.（从……到……）

他决定从天津开车到青岛。

from side to side　The monkey leaped from side to side.（从一边到另一边）

猴子从一边窜跳到另一边。

from time to time　She changed her teaching style from time to time.（不时地）

她时不时地变换一下教学风格。

G

gaze at　She gazed fixedly at the blue sky and remained motionless.（盯住，凝视）

她凝视着蓝天，一动不动。

get tired　Have some rest when you get tired.（疲倦，累了）

累了你就休息一下。

◆除非身体非常健康并且没有任何毒素与紧张，否则一个舒适的姿势是不易做到的。

H

have difficulty (in) doing   He has difficulty bending forward.（做某事有困难）

他前屈很困难。

I

if necessary   I can translate that article for you if necessary.（如果必要的话）

如果必要的话，我可以为你翻译那篇文章。

if possible   If possible, you may close your eyes while holding the pose.（如果可以的话）

如果可以的话，你可以在保持这个体式的时候闭上眼睛。

in a straight line   The teacher required us to stand in a straight line.（在一条直线上）

老师要求我们站成一条直线。

in alignment with   Check that your hands are in alignment with your feet.（与……成一条直线）

确保你的双手与双脚处于一条直线上。

in and out   There are actually many ways in and out.（进进出出）

实际上有许多条路能进进出出。

in contact with   His fingertips were in contact with the floor for support.（与……接触）

他的手指指尖接触地板作为支撑。

◆ Purity of heart and equanimity of mind are the very essence of Yoga.

in front of   You can park your car in front of our yoga studio next time.
（在……前面）

下次你可以把车停在我们瑜伽馆前面。

in line with   See that your head is in line with your neck and spine.
（在一条直线上）

确保你的头与颈部、脊柱在一条直线上。

in one's mind   You should keep these key points in your mind.（在某人的头脑中）

你应当记住这些要点。

in the back of   He came late so that he had no choice but to practise in the back of the classroom.（在……的后面）

他来晚了，因此别无选择，只能到教室后面练习。

in case of   Call this number in case of emergency.（如果发生）

遇到紧急情况就打这个电话。

in the air   I feel as if I am flying in the air.（在空中）

我感到自己好像在空中飞翔。

in the present   Most people do not know how to live in the present.
（现在）

大多数人不知道如何活在当下。

in the world   An unknown virus was spreading in the world when the winter holiday started.（在世界上）

寒假刚开始的时候，一种未知的病毒正在世界各地传播。

◆心地纯洁和头脑平静是瑜伽的精髓。

instead of You should stop there instead of forcing yourself to go deeper into the pose.（而不是）

你应该停在那里，而不是强迫自己更深入体式。

It is more...to do...than to do...

It is more interesting to go hiking than to stay indoors.（比起……做……更……）

去远足比待在家里有趣得多。

It's time to It's time to review what I've learned in today's class.（是……的时候）

是时候复习一下我在今天课堂中学到的东西了。

K

keep alert Try to keep alert during the practice.（保持警觉）

练习过程中尽量保持警觉。

keep...in place Keep your hands in place and jump back.（保持……在适当位置）

保持双手固定不动，向后跳。

L

let go Concentrate on your breath and let go of everything.（放开，释放）

关注你的呼吸，放开一切。

let loose She let her hair loose and it fell around her shoulders.（让……自由，释放，放开）

她的头发一解开，便顺着肩膀垂了下来。(p.1197)

◆ Lead a dedicated life. That way you experience the divine in yourself.

lie down Lie down on a flat surface and relax.（躺下）

躺在一个平面上，放松。

lie on one's abdomen/stomach

Lie on your abdomen, and rest for a few minutes.（俯卧）

俯卧下来，休息几分钟。

line up You had better line your car up with the ones that have already been parked there.（对齐）

你最好让你的车和那些已经停在那里的车对齐。

look ahead Stand upright and look straight ahead.（向前看）

站直，直视前方。

look down Look down and check the position of your feet.（向下看）

低头检查你双脚的位置。

look over You can twist your neck to look over a shoulder.（从……上面看）

你可以转动颈部从肩膀上方看过去。

look up Look up and feel the stretch in the front of your neck.（抬头看，向上看）

向上看，感受颈部前侧的拉伸。

loosen up Rotate your shoulders to loosen up tight muscles.〔放松（肌肉）〕

转动肩膀以放松僵紧的肌肉。

M

make it easy   You can introduce variations and make it easy for students to follow your instructions in yoga class. （使其变得容易）

你可以引入变体，让学生在瑜伽课上轻松跟上你的口令。

make sure (that)   Make sure you do not fall asleep in meditation. （确保）

确保自己不在冥想时睡着。

move into   They will move into a new house next week. （进入）

下周他们将搬进新房子。

move on to   Okay, I think we could move on to the next topic. 〔开始做（别的事），移到〕

好，我想咱们可以进行下一个话题了。

N

next to   He sat next to her. （紧挨着）

他紧挨着她坐下。

not at all   What the teacher said was not at all clear. （一点也不）

老师说的一点都不清楚。

O

one at a time   You can only type in the customers' information one at a time. （一次一个）

你一次只能输入一个客户的信息。

◆ Why worry what others say of you? You should know who you are.

one by one　His friends left him one by one when he was in trouble.
（一个接一个，逐一）

当他遇到麻烦时，他的朋友一个接一个地离他而去。

on the other side　The grass is always greener on the other side of the
fence.（在另一边）

篱笆外的草总是更加绿（喻指这山望着那山高）。

on top of　Yoga blocks were piled on top of one another.（在……之上）

瑜伽砖一块摞一块地堆在一起。

opposite to　He sat opposite to her.（与……相反，在……对面）

他坐在她对面。

P

perpendicular to　Make sure your arms and legs are perpendicular to
the floor.（垂直于）

确保你的双臂和双腿垂直于地板。

place...on...　Place your hands on your abdomen.（把……放在……上）

将你的双手放在腹部上。

press against　Your inner knees press against the mat.（挤压，压
在……上）

让你的双膝内侧压在垫子上。

press...into...　Press your hands firmly into the floor.（迫使，强迫）

将你的双手牢牢地压向地板。

put...on...　Could you please put the bolster on that shelf?（放）

请把抱枕放到那个架子上好吗？

◆为什么要担心别人怎么说你？你应该知道你是谁。

R

raise up　He raised himself up on one elbow.（举起，抬起）

他用一只胳膊肘支起身子。

relative to　Is the position of the sun relative to the earth changing all time?（相对于）

太阳和地球的相对位置一直在发生变化吗？

relax into　Relax into the soft music and enjoy it.（因放松下来而转入……）

在柔和的音乐中放松并享受它。

remember to　Please remember to open all the windows when you arrive.（记得）

在你到达后，请记得打开所有窗户。

rest...against...　Rest your back against the wall.（靠着）

让你的后背靠在墙上。

rest on　Your hands may rest on your belly.（停留在，被搁在）

你的双手可以放在腹部上。

return to　Return to Tadasana and relax with your eyes closed.（回到）

回到山式站立，闭上双眼放松。

rise and fall　You have no other choice but to accept the rise and fall of your life.（涨落，起落）

你别无选择，只能接受生活的起起落落。

rising and falling　Focus on your breath and feel the rising and falling of your abdomen.（升降，起伏）

关注你的呼吸，感受腹部的起伏。

◆ To weigh the ego, just take a long piece of paper and pencil and list all that you call yours: your name, your fame, your position, your power, your brain—everything. If your list is long, you really carry a heavy load.

rush to Get up early and you don't have to rush to work.（着急做，匆匆赶往）

早起你就不用赶着去上班了。

S

see that... Please see that you turn off the lights before you leave.（注意，务必，确保）

确保离开之前把灯关掉。

sense of balance Tree pose can help you create a sense of balance.（平衡感）

树式能够帮你建立起平衡感。

settle down In the beginning, it might take quite a while for your mind to settle down.（安定下来，平静下来）

刚开始的时候，可能需要很长一段时间才能让你的头脑平静下来。

shift...to... Shift your weight to your right foot.（转向）

将你的身体重心转移到右脚上。

sit down Sit down, please.（坐下）

请坐下。

sit up He had to sit up and drink some water to suppress his cough.（端坐，坐直身子）

他不得不坐起来喝点水止住咳嗽。

so that Lift your spine up towards the ceiling so that your torso is perpendicular to the floor.〔（引出结果）因此，所以〕

将你的脊柱向天花板上提，这样一来，你的躯干便会垂

◆要衡量自我，只需拿出长纸条和铅笔，列出所有你称之为自己的东西：你的名字、你的名声、你的地位、你的权力、你的大脑——一切。如果你的清单很长，那么你的负担真的很重。

直于地板。

start from   We will start from the basic postures.（从……开始）

我们会从基础体式开始。

state of mind   She went into a whole new state of mind by practising

meditation.（心境，心理状态）

通过练习冥想，她进入到一种全新的心理状态。

stay awake   I turned up the volume to stay awake.（保持清醒）

我把音量调大来保持清醒。

stop doing   Please stop talking when you enter the room.（停止

做……）

当你进到房间的时候，请停止交谈。

stretch out   Stretch out your legs and arms.（伸出）

伸出你的双腿和双臂。

such as   You can use different props such as yoga strap and block.（例如）

你可以使用不同的辅具，如瑜伽伸展带和瑜伽砖。

suffer from   He has been suffering from depression for several years.

（患……病，遭受）

他患抑郁症有好多年了。

T

take...down   Can you take the clock down from the wall for me?（拿下）

你能帮我把墙上的钟表拿下来吗？

take hold of   Take hold of the outsides of your feet.（抓住，握着）

抓住你脚的外侧。

◆ If you can make your mind pure, then the whole world is your friend.

take its course Relax and let everything take its course.（任其自然
发展）

放松，让一切顺其自然吧！

talk to Please feel free to talk to me when you are in trouble.（与……
交谈）

当你有困难时请随时跟我讲。

the other Sometimes you may find one leg is more flexible than the
other one.（另一个，其他的）

有时候你会感觉自己的一条腿比另一条腿更灵活些。

the other way around She has sacrificed a lot for him, and not the
other way around.（反过来，倒过来）

她为他牺牲了很多，而不是相反。

the same with It's the same with what you experienced last night.
（与……一样）

这和你昨晚经历的一样。

There is... There is a dog over there.〔有（表示存在）〕

那儿有一条狗。

too...to... I am too hungry to continue working.（太……以至不能）

我太饿了，不能继续工作了。

to start with To start with, you have to have the courage to stand on
the yoga mat.（首先）

首先，你得有勇气站到垫子上。

try to He tried not to laugh at this moment.（试着，努力，设法）

他忍着不在此刻笑出来。

◆如果你能让自己的思想纯洁，那么整个世界都是你的朋友。

U

under the supervision of Beginners should practise yoga under the supervision of a qualified teacher. （在······的监督下）

初学者应当在有资质的老师的监督指导下练习瑜伽。

use...as... Sun Salutation can be used as warming-up for advanced practitioners. （把······当作······使用）

高级练习者可以用拜日式作为热身。

use...to... Use your breath to release the tightness in the back of your legs. （使用）

用呼吸来释放你腿部后面的紧张感。

W

with the help of You can make much more progress with the help of a professional teacher. （在······的帮助下）

在专业老师的帮助下，你可以取得更大的进步。